THE CLINICIAN'S GUIDE TO LINGUISTIC
LANGUAGE IMPAIRMENT

Far Communication Disorders Series

Series Editors: Chris Code and David Rowley, Department of Speech Pathology, Leicester Polytechnic, Leicester, England.

The *Far Communication Disorders Series* aims to provide books in speech and language pathology and therapy for the clinician and student clinician. Each book in the series will aim to be practical, readable and affordable. Currently available and forthcoming titles include:

Parents, Families, and the Stuttering Child
Edited by Lena Rustin

Treating Phonological Disorders in Children. Metaphon - Theory to Practice
Janet Howell & Elizabeth Dean

Assessment and Management of Emotional and Psychosocial Reactions to Aphasia and Brain Damage
Peter Währborg

Group Encounters in Communication Disorders
Edited by Margaret Fawcus

Management of Acquired Aphasia in Children
Janet Lees

The Clinician's Guide to Linguistic Profiling of Language Impairment
Martin J Ball

Cluttering: A Clinical Perspective
Edited by Florence Myers & Kenneth O St Louis

Computers in Management and Therapy
Edited by David Rowley & Chris Code

Introductory Guide to Clinical Syntactic Analysis
Eeva Leinonen & Susan Fasler

Which Screen? A User's Guide to Speech and Language Screening Tests
Joanne Corcoran

Far Communication Disorders Series

THE CLINICIAN'S GUIDE
TO LINGUISTIC PROFILING
OF LANGUAGE IMPAIRMENT

Martin J Ball
University of Ulster

Far Communications
Kibworth

Copyright 1992 by **Far Communications Ltd.,**
5 Harcourt Estate, Kibworth, Leics. LE8 0NE,
Great Britain (Tel. 0533 796166)

British Library Cataloguing in Publication Data:

Ball, Martin J
  Clinician's Guide to Linguistic
  Profiling of Language Impairment. - (Far
  Communication Disorders Series)
  I. Title II. Series
  616.85

  ISBN 0-9514728-8-7

Printed and Bound in Great Britain

CONTENTS

Preface   v

Chapter 1   1
Profiles
    1.1 Tests and Profiles
    1.2 Levels of analysis
    1.3 Phonetics and Phonology
    1.4 Morphology and Syntax
    1.5 Lexis and Semantics
    1.6 Pragmatics and Sociolinguistics

Chapter 2   11
Phonetics
    2.1 Articulation tests
    2.2 Phonetic transcription of disordered speech

Chapter 3   23
Segmental Phonology
    3.1 PROPH
    3.2 PACS
    3.3 Other Profiles

Chapter 4   45
Suprasegmental Phonology
    4.1 PROP
    4.2 PROVOQ

Chapter 5   55
Morphology and Syntax
    5.1 Morpheme analysis
    5.2 LARSP
    5.3 ASS/CSD
    5.4 Other Profiles

Chapter 6   75
Semantics
    6.1 PRISM-G
    6.2 PRISM-L

Chapter 7   95
Pragmatics
    7.1 Pragmatic Protocol
    7.2 PCA
    7.3 Other Profiles

Chapter 8   103
Sociolinguistics and Bilingualism
    8.1 Sociolinguistics
    8.2 Bilingualism

References   117

Index   125

PREFACE

In the last fifteen years or so we have witnessed a growth in a new kind of assessment tool in the speech-language pathology clinic: the linguistic profile. Whereas previously emphasis in assessment was on standardized testing, the profile eschewed both numerical scoring and the selective elicitation procedures adopted by most such tests. As devised initially by Crystal and his colleagues, the profile set out to use a representative sample of the patient's speech to provide a picture of that patient's linguistic abilities and disabilities. Instead of a numerical scoring procedure, profiles often offered a metric based on developmental norms; and instead of a pass-fail result, the profile was able to point directly at the structures that needed remediation, and the order in which this should be undertaken.

Over the period of the development of such an approach to assessment, we have seen profiles devised in most areas of linguistic analysis. While LARSP, dealing with syntax, was the first developed, we now have profiles in phonology - both segmental and suprasegmental, semantics, pragmatics, and socio- linguistics. The recent growth in provision of profiles at all levels of analysis means that we have to take a selective approach in this book. We have included accounts of the most influential profiles at the levels of phonology, syntax and semantics, and selected two representative profiles in the field of pragmatics - an area relatively new to speech-language pathology. Nevertheless, we have also attempted to include information on older, or less well-known profiles, and on attempts to computerize profiles in the respective chapters.

As well as the above areas of linguistic analysis, we also include chapters on phonetics, and in particular the recent developments in the transcription of disordered speech, and on sociolinguistics and bilingualism where, although little formal work exists on profiles, their importance to adequate linguistic assessment cannot be underestimated.

I would like to thank Chris Code for giving me the

opportunity of writing this book, and putting up with the continual changes in submission date. I also want to express my grateful thanks to Tom Powell for providing me with so much information on assessment techniques in the United States.

Martin J. Ball
December 1991.

Acknowledgements

We would like to thank the following for permission to reproduce the profile charts included in this book: Professor David Crystal for the following profile forms: PROPH, PROP, LARSP, PRISM-L, PRISM-G; NFER-Nelson for certain charts from PACS; Claire Penn for the PCA chart; Diane Kirchner for the Pragmatic Protocol.

Chapter 1

PROFILES

1.1 Tests and Profiles

Over the last fifteen years or so, the use of linguistic profiles in the assessment of speech-language impairments has grown considerably. This has, to some extent, been at the expense of more traditional assessment procedures such as standardized tests. We have not the space here to explore in detail the advantages that have been claimed for profiles over quantitative testing (such arguments are explored in some depth in Crystal, Fletcher and Garman, 1976 and in Müller, Munro and Code, 1981), but we will take a little time to look at the differences between the two approaches.

Quantitative testing is generally standardized on a representative sample of normal speakers (children or adults or both, depending on the target population of the test). This means that the scores assigned for particular areas of a test are calculated so that "average" or "acceptable" scores are directly relatable to what the standardized population would produce on average.

A further feature of most tests of this sort is the fact that they generally concentrate on particular aspects of speech or language. For example, articulation tests often require the tester to transcribe particular consonants or consonant clusters (only rarely are vowels included) in a set of test words uttered once only by the subject.

Finally, we must bear in mind what a test gives us: a score. This may be very useful in an initial assessment to let us know whether a client does or does not fall broadly into the category of speech-language impaired, however it often cannot tell us much more. By this we mean that scores often obscure which part of the client's phonology, or syntax etc. is actually impaired: the knowledge of which is naturally vital if we are going to be able

1

to plan an effective programme of remediation.

So, standardized quantitative tests are generally selective in the material that is investigated - leading to the lack of a comprehensive picture of the client's abilities; they rely too much on the record of single responses to test requirements in an often very abnormal communicative situation; and by presenting the clinician with a numerical score they can only aid in basic questions of client classification, but not with more detailed diagnoses nor with the development of treatment plans.

The aim of a linguistic profile is to provide an assessment tool that avoids these drawbacks. An ideal profile should, therefore, be comprehensive rather than selective; it should be derived from natural speech, including spontaneous speech wherever possible, and where all occurrences of a token are analysed; and should present as a "result" an overall picture of the client's performance (from which we can infer their abilities and impairments), allowing a principled planning of intervention strategies.

Crystal (1982) defines a profile as follows "a linguistic profile is a principled description of just those features of a person's... use of language which will enable him (sic) to be identified for a specific purpose" (p1). The use of the term "principled" implies that the linguistic data are to be analysed according to an agreed theoretical framework, be they phonological, syntactic or of any other type. We will return to this in the consideration of the specific profiles described in following chapters.

We must also consider the phrase "use of language". As we have already noted, one of the weaknesses claimed for traditional tests has been that they have not investigated a client's use of language adequately. Most people working with profiles have stressed the need to gain representative data from patients. This means that the use of picture naming tasks or similar standardized methods of data elicitation are to be avoided, or at least should not be the sole method of gaining access to the speaker's linguistic repertoire. Rather, profiles lay emphasis on the recording of spontaneous speech on the one hand, and the use of questions and answers to promote conversational exchanges on the other.

Tests look for short easy to manage utterances; profiles look for longer, data-rich utterances.

We see, then, that profiles often suggest that a relatively long period of speech (say, half-an-hour) should be tape-recorded, and all of it transcribed and/or analysed, and then put on to the profile chart. This amount of data normally guarantees that most categories in the system will occur, and the most common will occur several times, allowing the analyst to investigate any inconsistent usages lost in the traditional test.

Profiles normally consist of charts which are divided into categories (e.g. syntactic categories, or phonological units), allowing the clinician to note how many times a particular category was used and, where appropriate, whether the category was utilized correctly or otherwise. Some profiles have an added dimension to aid in the classification of patients. This has most normally been a developmental metric (e.g. LARSP, PACS), whereby the patient can be assessed in terms of what level of normal linguistic development they have reached in comparison with their actual age.

This book is an attempt to provide clinicians with a guide to the use of profiles, and naturally individual profiles have different instructions for use. Nevertheless, the profiles we examine below are all based on the principles outlined above. However, although profiles claim to be comprehensive, they can only in fact be comprehensive within one particular level of linguistic analysis: otherwise they would simply be too complicated to complete or to read. In the next section we will examine what is meant be a "level of linguistic analysis", how many such levels are generally recognized, and what they are.

1.2 Levels of Analysis

Language is a complex, multi-layered symbol system whereby aspects of the real world are realized as a series of noises produced in the human vocal tract. By multi-layered we mean that speech sounds can be grouped into phonemes (contrastive sounds), and then into syllables; these in turn are grouped into morphemes (meaningful word components), then words; which in turn are

3

grouped into phrases, clauses and sentences which finally convey meaning.

Linguists have therefore approached the analysis of speech and language in terms of levels, as to do otherwise would produce analyses too complicated to read. Traditionally, linguists have ordered the levels of analysis from speech through to meaning (though others have utilised the opposite ordering). These levels are normally termed phonetics, phonology, morphology, syntax, lexis and semantics; these will be described briefly in turn as they correspond directly to the following chapters.

1.3 Phonetics and Phonology
These two terms both refer to the sounds of language (i.e. speech), but while they have this in common it is important not to confuse phonetics and phonology as the difference between them is not only important theoretically, but also in terms of language disorders and remediation. Whereas phonetics is the study of speech sounds irrespective of their function in language, (see Chapter 2) phonology is the study of how speech sounds function in language.

We can give an example to clarify this distinction: an analysis of all the speech sounds produced by a patient during a representative sample of speech would give us **phonetic** data. However, unless we know the function of those speech sounds in the target language, we will not be able to say whether the sounds marked incorrect will actually interfere with comprehension: in other words we need a **phonological** analysis of the data as well.

If an RP (= "received pronunciation" or standard middle class speech) British English patient, for example, produces vowels of the type [a], [e], [o] where we might have expected [æ], [eɪ] and [əʊ], we could well classify these as "phonetic errors"; however if a phonological analysis shows that the expected RP vowels are consistently replaced by the phones noted above which in turn never occur elsewhere, then the function of the expected set has been taken over directly by the new set, and no confusion in comprehension will occur; at worst the patient will sound like a northern British English speaker.

Let us take another example from English. The English "l" sound has two main variants: the so-called "clear l" and "dark l". The clear l occurs, for example, in the word "leaf" and is transcribed phonetically as [l]; the dark l occurs, for example, in the word "feel" and is transcribed phonetically as [ɫ]. These two separate sounds (or "phones") are, however, in *complementary distribution* in most accents of English: that is to say that clear l occurs in positions in words where dark l never occurs, and vice versa. Because they are phonetically so similar, and because they are in complementary distribution most speakers consider them to be simply a single sound type, that is "l". Phonology recognizes this type of relation between sounds, so we say that English has one **phoneme** /l/, consisting of two **allophones**: [l] before vowels, and [ɫ] after vowels and after consonants at the end of syllables. This kind of analysis is language-specific, however, as clear and dark l may be separate phonemes (i.e. be capable of distinguishing one word from another) in some languages, or one (or both) types of l may be absent from a language altogether.

Now this grouping of (allo)phones into phonemes is important also for the clinical linguist. Taking our example of /l/ again, a patient who confuses the allophones [l] and [ɫ] is going to sound odd, but will still be understood; whereas a patient who confuses /l/ with /r/ is likely to cause comprehension difficulties. This is because /l/ and /r/ are separate phonemes (as shown by the slant brackets //) which distinguish words (e.g. "lead" - "red", "mallow" - "marrow", etc.), whereas [l] and [ɫ] cannot be used to distinguish one word from another as they can never occur in the same phonetic environment.

However, the study of phonology is not simply a matter of working out from phonetic data what are the phonemes of a language (or indeed the phonological units used by a speaker with disordered speech). Phonologists have noted phonological processes involving whole sets of phonemes when they are found in particular environments. Ideas like these can be very helpful in clinical phonology, in working out the relationship between the target sound(s) of the language and what a patient actually

5

produces. We return to notions like these in Chapter 3. It must also be remembered that phonology can be investigated at both the level of the single segment (or phoneme) (see Chapter 3), but also at a higher level, across segments, (as in intonation) (see Chapter 4); and that these need to be investigated separately for each patient.

What is needed in any assessment of the speech of a patient is an approach that combines both the phonetic level and the phonological level. Any analysis that ignores fine phonetic detail is in danger of assigning sounds to the wrong category and thereby giving a false impression of a patient's abilities; while an approach that looks only at phonetics ignores the fact that sounds are used in language, and used differentially.

1.4 Morphology and Syntax

These two levels of analysis are often grouped together under the term "grammar" (although some linguists use "grammar" with a different meaning). Both levels are concerned with the structure of language (as opposed to speech): morphology with word structure, syntax with sentence structure.

The main unit of word structure that is used in linguistics is the **morpheme**. This is usually defined as being the smallest unit of linguistic structure that is meaning bearing. Thus "dog" is one morpheme, for although we can break it down into individual phonemes (contrastive sounds), we cannot break it down into smaller units that bear any kind of meaning. On the other hand "beautifully", although a single word, can be broken down into smaller units that have some kind of meaning attached to them: "beauty" + "ful" +"ly", where the first unit represents the concept, the second (the adjectival ending) alters the meaning to a descriptive word for things that possess the original concept, and the third unit (the adverbial ending) alters the meaning to a descriptive word for actions or states possessing the concept.

We have seen so far, then, that some morphemes can stand alone as single words (like "dog"); these are termed **free morphemes**. Others (like "ful" and "ly") can only occur when attached to other morphemes; these are termed **bound morphemes**.

6

Very often in English bound morphemes act as "extra" bits of meaning attached to the basic part of a word; in these cases their function is one of **affixes** (**prefixes** at the beginning of a word, and **suffixes** at the end), while the main part of the word is termed the **root**. The term **stem** is also found: this refers to that part of a word excluding the particular affix under consideration, so it may be a root, or a root plus one or more affixes.

Further, affixes can be seen to be of two main types in English. One type has grammatical function, in that the "meaning" associated with them is largely to do with grammatical features such as number, tense and so on. Examples include the -s ending of English regular plurals and -ed ending of regular past tenses. This kind of affix is termed an **inflectional affix**, and words with these affixes are considered simply variants of the basic word. The other type is one that is considered to create a new word, either by changing the class of a word, or by creating a new word of the same class. Examples include the "-ful" ending we saw above, or the "-ness" ending of "happiness", or the "un-" prefix of "unhappy", etc. This type of affix is termed a **derivational affix**.

This distinction is important for both language development and for disordered language. This is because it appears that whereas as words with derivational affixes are learnt as whole new words rather than as a word to which something has been added in the majority of cases, the opposite seems to happen with inflectional affixes. Here, the affixes are learnt to be used with one or two words and then eventually their usage is generalised across the board, and so they become used with all words in a particular word class. We can therefore chart the chronological development of inflectional affixes. Likewise in disordered language, we may find that inflectional affixes are omitted, or used wrongly, but this is not often the case with derivational affixes. We will see in Chapter 5 that, where morphology is assessed in profiles, it is inflectional morphology that is looked at, not derivational.

Syntax, as we noted above, is the study of sentence structure. This isn't simply the analysis of the order of words in a sentence, though it is important to know what order constituents of sentences normally occur in, and what constituents (if any) have the freedom to occur in more than one order for emphasis purposes and so on.

One of the main objectives of syntax is to indentify the hierarchy of constituents that a sentence is made up of. By this we mean to see what are the main grammatical roles that we find in a sentence, what types of word or word-groups can be found as making up these roles, and what relations (or morphology (i.e. affixes), or syntax, in this instance word-ordering) hold between them.

Let us give examples. Traditionally, the main syntactic roles are termed subject, verb, object, complement and adverbial (some grammarians use different terms, but these are probably the most widely known). Brief definitions of these roles are that Subject is the role controlling the action or state of the sentence grammatically, verb refers to the action or state, object is the role that the action or state controls, complement is a role that shares an identity with a previous subject or object, and adverbial is a role grammatically loosely linked to the other roles with, usually, an ability to appear in various places within the sentence.

The grammatical link between the subject and the verb is seen in English in two ways: morphologically some subject types require particular verb endings in some tenses (e.g. "I run" - "she runs"), and syntactically in that in declarative sentences the subject comes before the verb. Examples of the other roles are given in Chapter 5.

The hierarchical nature of syntactic analysis is taken further when we examine in detail one particular role: in this case the subject. If we ask what word classes or constituents can fill this sentence slot, we find quite a long list: for example, a pronoun, a noun, an adjective plus a noun, a determiner (e.g. "the", "a") plus a noun, a determiner plus an adjective plus a noun, and numerous others.

It is clear, then, that any syntactic analysis of either normal or disordered language is a complex activity which must be carried out thoroughly if we are to find out what someone's syn-

8

tactic capabilities really are. Further, it is also obvious that such a complex system cannot be learnt by a child as a complete system: indeed research shows that specific parts of the system are acquired in a set order. This means that a knowledge of syntactic development in normal children can be used as a guide to the assessment of patients with syntactic disorders.

1.5 Lexis and Semantics

Lexis is the term linguists use to describe the study of vocabulary. The term **lexeme** is often encountered as alternative to the ambiguous term "word". A lexeme is a vocabulary item which encompasses all those variants brought about through the addition (or otherwise) of inflectional affixes (see the discussion on morphology above). So, *walk, walks, walking, walked* are all considered part of one lexeme, but *happy, happiness* and *unhappy* are considered three lexemes (because the differences come about through the addition of derivational affixes).

Both in normal language development, and in clinical linguistics, we often encounter descriptions of the size of a speaker's vocabulary. We must always be aware that such information is more usually expressed in lexemes rather than words, and that is the method adopted in the main profile of lexis described in Chapter 6.

However, a simple description of numbers of lexemes is not very helpful. The purpose of lexemes (and, of course, of language as a whole) is semantic: to express meaning. It is more useful, then, to list lexemes in terms of their semantic fields, that is the different areas of meaning. In that way we can see if a patient is able to express themselves well in a particular area of meaning, but may lack lexemes in another area.

Meaning is not restricted to the lexical aspects of language, however. In sentences we can identify not only syntactic roles (see section 1.4 above), but also semantic ones. These include roles such as **actor**, **activity** and **goal**, that often correspond to syntactic roles such as subject, verb and object. Notions of grammatical or sentence semantics are explored more fully in Chapter 6.

1.6 Pragmatics and Sociolinguistics

There are numerous other areas of language study that linguists have pursued, but in terms of clinical linguistics we can identify two main areas of importance: pragmatics and sociolinguistics.

It is not always easy to draw a distinction between these two areas, particularly as there are no universally accepted definitions of them (particularly so with pragmatics). As a working distinction we can say that whereas both pragmatics and sociolinguistics are to do with the interaction between language and extra-linguistic features, pragmatics concentrates on the contexts of language usage, while sociolinguistics concentrates on the interaction between social variables and speakers' use of language (there are several areas of study that have been "claimed" by both disciplines).

For clinical linguistics the areas of pragmatics most of interest, perhaps, are aspects such as discourse (conversation) strategies - both between therapist and patient, and between patient and other speakers; non-verbal communication, such as the use of gesture and posture; and speech act behaviour, such as the ability to persuade or argue. We will see in Chapter 7 how pragmatic behaviour has become the focus of profile designers in recent times.

A clinical sociolinguistics is perhaps a less developed area. Sociolinguists have examined the interaction between class membership, sex, regional background, ethnic background, age and other topics and the use of language varieties. It has also encompassed the study of bilingualism. All these areas are of interest to the clinician, but as yet few attempts have been made to profile such a large area of language use. Nevertheless, in Chapter 8 we look in more detail at sociolinguistics (and in particular, bilingualism) and how we might attempt examine this information in language assessment.

Chapter 2

PHONETICS

Introduction

As noted in Chapter 1, any assessment of a patient's speech (as opposed to language) requires an analysis of both the phonetics and phonology. A phonetic analysis alone will not tell us how a patient uses the sounds described, but an adequate phonological analysis cannot be constructed without detailed phonetic data to work on. Indeed, many of the so-called "articulation tests" are not in fact detailed analyses of a patient's articulation at all, but ask only for a superficial and overly abstract phonological transcription of the patient's speech (see criticisms in Müller, Munro and Code, 1981).

We must also bear in mind that speech can not only be looked at in terms of the distinction between phonetic form and phonological function, but also between the segmental and suprasegmental approaches. By this we mean that phoneticians have traditionally worked with the idea that much of the speech signal can be reduced to sound segments (although in reality this is somewhat simplistic in that boundaries between such sound segments are not always easy to describe). These sound segments are what we identify in phonetic transcription as separate phones requiring separate symbols, and on a phonological level we can often group such phones into phonemes (the minimal units of sound having a contrastive function: that is capable of distinguishing one word from another), phonemes being thought of phonologically as individual segments.

However, there is also much important phonetic information that can not be reduced to the segmental level, as it occurs over several segments. This information is termed "suprasegmental" (= over segments), or "prosodic" information. Like all phonetic data, this too can be reduced to functional, or contrastive, units, and so can be described in both phonetic and phonological terms. The suprasegmental phonetic information most usually described by phoneticians includes length, stress, pitch (as intonation), voice quality, loudness and tempo. All these features may be subject to disruption in speech disordered patients, so just as much as segmental phonology, we need to be able to profile aspects of disordered prosody. These aspects are returned to in Chapter 3.

We have talked about the necessity of good phonetic data, which raises the question of how we record such information. We can of course use instrumental means (see for example Code and Ball, 1984), but while this is important for detailed studies, it is often not feasible for everyday clinical usage. Phonetic transcription using the alphabet of the International Phonetic Association (IPA) is the recommended way of capturing patients' speech output for analysis. It is recommended that this is done from audio or video recordings, as live transcriptions often miss much information, and will interfere with clinician-patient interaction. The IPA in its most recent revision (1989) now provides a set of symbols and diacritics especially designed for the transcription of the sorts of rare or non-normal sounds encountered in disordered speech (see Duckworth, Allen, Hardcastle and Ball, 1990), and these are to be recommended over clinicians' own ad hoc inventions, as these last will obviously be opaque to other researchers trying to read such transcriptions. Further details of these symbols are given below, and the complete IPA alphabet, together with the Extensions for Disordered Speech, is included at the end of this chapter.

2.1 Articulation tests

We noted above that the traditional method of acquiring data for speech (as opposed to language) analysis has been through the "articulation test". Probably the most commonly used articulation test in Britain is the "Edinburgh Articulation Test" (EAT: Anthony, Bogle, Ingram and McIsaac, 1971), and in the US is the "Goldman-Fristoe Test of Articulation" (GFTA: Goldman and Fristoe, 1972).

We have already noted that these articulation tests are, in fact, not phonetic in purpose, but phonological. The name therefore is something of a misnomer. We deal with them here, however, as they provide guidelines for the collection of (phonetic) data, as well as for its analysis.

The data collection procedures of both tests are similar (though the GFTA does also allow the use of spontaneous speech). These involve the production by the patient of a small set. of lexical items from pictures presented by the clinician. The lexical items are designed to contain a representative sample of the phonemes of the language (i.e. English in the case of these two tests) in various positions within the word (i.e. word-initial, word-medial, word-final). The tester listens to the performance of the patient (which is usually tape-recorded of course), and transcribes the sound made by the patient for the target in the test word. These responses can later by graded as to whether they were the same as the target, phonetically different from the target but not confusable with another phoneme of English ("distort-ions"), phonetically different from the target to such an extent that the sound is confusable with another phoneme of English ("substitution"), or the sound is left out ("omission"). In this way, an overall score can be arrived at for each patient, compared with standardized scores obtained from representative samples of normal speakers, and the clincian can see whether a phonological problem exists for a particular patient.

There are, however, numerous problems with this approach: both to do with data acquisition and data analysis. As noted above, the GFTA does allow the use of spontaneous as well as elicited speech to be analysed, and it can be argued that the EAT also can be applied to speech samples obtained in other ways. Nevertheless, both tests do encourage the use of picture elicitation to provide the core data for the analysis. It is a quick method of obtaining a wide sample of phoneme types, so what exactly is wrong with it?

Firstly, it is not natural. We do not normally speak in single word utterances in response to the showing of a picture. We normally speak multi-word utterances in response to some verbal stimulus from a conversational partner, or as a verbal stimulus to such a partner. In other words, except for those patients who are normally restricted to very short utterances, the type of speech elicited is not representative of most speakers.

There is a further problem to such short utterances. Phonological effects (called "co-articulations") that take place across word-boundaries cannot be explored via such short speech samples. In may well be that a patient's phonological behaviour for certain sounds will depend upon the phonological environment of neighbouring words: single word elicitation tests cannot take this into account.

Thirdly, the construction of many articulation tests into three phonological places: word-initial, word-medial and word-final, has been criticized by, for example, Grunwell (1985). Grunwell makes the point that the medial position (in English at any rate) consists, in reality, of two separate positions dependant on the syllable boundary: syllable-initial word-medial and syllable-final word-medial (compare *bee|keeper* vs *beef|eater*). Phonological processes such as the deletion of syllable-final consonants may well operate word-medially, but only on those consonants that are syllable-final and word-medial.

Further to this is the problem that the phonemes are tested in each position only once, and perhaps also in consonant clusters. So for /p/, the EAT tests this phoneme in the following words: *pencil, sleeping, spoon, stamps*. It is well known that patients with disordered phonologies often demonstrate considerable variability, especially during treatment where correct and incorrect forms of a phoneme may occur in an apparently random way. If we test a sole example of initial /p/, we may lose the fact that that sound might have a range of realizations.

Finally, we have to consider the scoring of tests such as these. While they undoubtedly give information that a particular patient is showing phonological disorder, they do not always point directly to the patient's patterns of use, and so may not aid in planning remediation.

It is clear, then, that any assessment procedure that relies on such a small data base as that proposed in most articulation tests cannot hope to profile the linguistic area concerned accurately. It is for this reason, therefore, that we have repeatedly stressed the importance of acquiring a suitably large amount of spontaneous speech (where possible) from a patient to serve as the input to a profiling exercise. In the case of speech disorders it is of course vital that this speech sample is adequately transcribed (indeed, this is the case even if only an articulation test is being attempted). In the next section we will look at how such transcription should be undertaken.

2.2 Phonetic transcription of disordered speech

Phonetic transcription can be either live or from recorded material. In clinical situations it is often difficult, or impossible, to undertake any kind of live transcription while at the same time keeping the full attention and confidence of the patient. It is natural, therefore, that the bulk of clinical phonetic transcription is done from recorded material.

It has to be remembered, however, that transcribing from tape recorded speech (however good the quality) does not always allow one to make a complete record of the patient's utterances. There are various behaviours that can be lost in this medium. For example, the difference between a labio-dental and a bilabial fricative is difficult to hear on tape alone, even more so the difference between a dental and an interdental fricative. Also lost is the fairly common habit of "silent articulations", where a patient may prepare to make, for example, a target bilabial articulation, but then proceed to a following vowel without pronouncing the consonant.

All of these might have been captured if brief "live notes" were made during the session, perhaps by a clinical phonetician aiding the speech pathologist.

An alternative, which avoids some of the problems of audio tape, is to use video (preferably as well as high quality audio tape). The video playback will supply much of the visual cues not picked up on audio.

However the material is stored, it must eventually be transcribed phonetically to paper. This is done to serve as an input to the various phonological assessment techniques available, and to be readily available to other clincians if necessary. Most speech pathologists are trained in phonetic transcription, using the International Phonetic Alphabet (IPA) or its slightly variant form as used in the US. However, not all are trained in narrow phonetic transcription, or in the use of recently developed specialist symbols devised to cover non-normal speech sounds (i.e. sounds not occurring in any known natural language).

Unfortunately, many clinicians develop the habit of transcribing phonemically; that is to say using a symbol from the inventory of phoneme symbols for their variety of English that is nearest to the sound they hear. As noted in Chapter 1, it is important in clinical transcription that the maximum of phonetic detail is provided. If, for example [φ] is transcribed as [f] in a patient who realises all target /p/ sounds as [φ], but retains target /f/ as [f], then it will look like a complete merger of target /p/ and /f/ has taken place when clearly this is not the case. The patient in this example has in fact maintained a phonological contrast (though one that is phonetically very close), but a broad, phonemic transcription will suggest that the patient has, in fact, lost that phonological contrast.

It is not only the precise articulatory quality that has to be looked for in a clinical transcription. Prosodic elements, such as the length of a segment, can be important. In a study reported in Code and Ball (1982), it was noted that an apraxic was unable to utilize voicing in stops and fricatives; all such segments being voiceless. However, transcribing target /f/ and /v/ both as [f] hid the fact that the speaker was able to retain the length distinction holding between these sounds in normal speakers. Some sort of distinction was therefore retained, which could be captured through a transcription of [f:] and [f]. Other prosodic features, such as voice quality, loudness, speed of speech and pitch/intonation are also potentially very important.

A further problem naturally arises when sounds occur in the data that are not only non-English (or whichever language is being dealt with), but are sounds not normally occurring in natural language. A range of these may be found in clinical data, including reverse labio-dental (or "dentolabials"), linguo-labials, percussives, reiteration, and various types of nasal friction.

16

Duckworth *et al* (1990) and Ball (1991) both discuss the development of phonetic transcription for disordered speech. We can refer here to early attempts to provide specialist transcription systems for this area, e.g. Bush (1973, in Ingram 1976), Dalton and Hardcastle (1977), Shriberg and Kent (1982), PRDS (1980, 1983), and Vieregge (1987); and for voice Laver (1980). Some of these are illustrated in Ball (1991). Many of these systems do provide symbols for non-normal speech segments, but the first to do this in any principled way was PRDS. More recently, the IPA set up a committee to extend the alphabet to include symbols for non-normal speech. The resultant "Extensions to the IPA" was based to some extent on the PRDS symbols (and so supersedes them), but also included some of the prosodic features mentioned above.

These "Extensions" symbols are listed at the end of this chapter together with a current version of the main IPA chart. It is recommended that all clinicians working with disordered speech should use these symbols wherever possible in order that we can promote a common system of phonetic representation.

The special symbols themselves are divided into several sections. The first of these deals with segments not represented on the main IPA chart, and is further sub-divided into place of articulation (e.g. dentolabials and bidentals), manner of articulation (e.g. nareal fricatives and reiterated articulation), air stream (e.g. non-normal ingressive/egressive and silent articulation), and vocal fold activity (e.g. partial voicing/devoicing and pre-aspiration).

The second main section deals with indeterminacy. This is very useful for the clinician, and allows the representation of various degrees of certainty in the recognition of a segment. This ranges from the perception only of a segment with no further detail clear, to the marking of what is thought to be a specific segment, but noting a slight degree of doubt.

The third section has symbolisations for voice quality, based on phonatory activity (e.g. whisper, or creak), or articulatory features (e.g. palatal or labial voice quality). The symbols here can be used either for stretches of speech or for individual segments.

The final section of the "Extensions" covers other aspects of connected speech. These include pausing, where different lengths of pause can be symbolized, and loudness and rate of speech. As with the voice quality markings, stretches of speech of a particular loudness or speed can be marked off through the use of braces.

Clearly, no system can claim to be able to cover all the possible phonetic data that may occur in the clinical situation. Nevertheless, the "Extensions" go a long way towards this goal. They even provide (through the use of the asterisk) a method of noting sounds that are not otherwise provided for. It must also be recognized that narrow phonetic transcription is not an easy task, and readers may wish to consult Shriberg and Lof (1991) for an account of research into the reliability of such transcription.

Finally, we can note that to undertake profiles of disordered communication it is not always necessary to transcribe a patient's utterances phonetically. For a profile dealing with syntax and morphology, semantics, or pragmatics, a transcription of the data into normal orthography is usually all that is needed. Even a profile of a speaker's intonation patterns can utilise normal orthography, providing that the intonation contours themselves are added to this in some way (see Chapter 4). Nevertheless, it is clear that no clinician can hope to deal adequately with most speech disorders without a good grasp of phonetic transcription. It may well be that the recent developments in phonetic transcription reported above will prove a challenge to established clinicians, but eventually will establish their worth.

THE INTERNATIONAL PHONETIC ALPHABET (revised to 1989)

CONSONANTS

	Bilabial	Labiodental	Dental	Alveolar	Postalveolar	Retroflex	Palatal	Velar	Uvular	Pharyngeal	Glottal
Plosive	p b			t d		ʈ ɖ	c ɟ	k g	q ɢ		ʔ
Nasal	m	ɱ		n		ɳ	ɲ	ŋ	ɴ		
Trill	ʙ			r					ʀ		
Tap or Flap				ɾ		ɽ					
Fricative	ɸ β	f v	θ ð	s z	ʃ ʒ	ʂ ʐ	ç ʝ	x ɣ	χ ʁ	ħ ʕ	h ɦ
Lateral fricative				ɬ ɮ							
Approximant		ʋ		ɹ		ɻ	j	ɰ			
Lateral approximant				l		ɭ	ʎ	ʟ			
Ejective stop	p'			t'			c'	k'	q'		
Implosive	ɓ ɠ			ɗ			ʄ	ɠ ʛ	ʛ		

Where symbols appear in pairs, the one to the right represents a voiced consonant. Shaded areas denote articulations judged impossible.

DIACRITICS

̥ Voiceless	n̥ d̥	̤ More rounded	ɔ̹	ʷ Labialized	tʷ dʷ	̃ Nasalized	ẽ
̬ Voiced	s̬ t̬	̜ Less rounded	ɔ̜	ʲ Palatalized	tʲ dʲ	ⁿ Nasal release	dⁿ
ʰ Aspirated	tʰ dʰ	̟ Advanced	u̟	ˠ Velarized	tˠ dˠ	ˡ Lateral release	dˡ
̤ Breathy voiced	b̤ a̤	̠ Retracted	i̠	̴ Pharyngealized	tˤ dˤ	̚ No audible release	d̚
̰ Creaky voiced	b̰ a̰	̈ Centralized	ë	̴ Velarized or pharyngealized	ɫ		
̼ Linguolabial	t̼ d̼	̽ Mid centralized	ě	̝ Raised	e̝ (ɹ̝ = voiced alveolar fricative)		
̪ Dental	t̪ d̪	̘ Advanced Tongue Root	e̘	̞ Lowered	e̞ (β̞ = voiced bilabial approximant)		
̺ Apical	t̺ d̺	̙ Retracted Tongue Root	e̙	̩ Syllabic	n̩		
̻ Laminal	t̻ d̻	˞ Rhoticity	ə˞	̯ Non-syllabic	e̯		

The IPA alphabet.

VOWELS

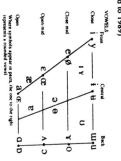

OTHER SYMBOLS

ʍ Voiceless labial-velar fricative
w Voiced labial-velar approximant
ɥ Voiced labial-palatal approximant
ʜ Voiceless epiglottal fricative
ʢ Voiced epiglottal fricative
ʡ Voiced epiglottal plosive
ɕ ʑ Alveolo-palatal fricatives
ɺ Alveolar lateral flap
ɧ Simultaneous ʃ and x

Affricates and double articulations can be represented by two symbols joined by a tie bar if necessary: k͡p t͡s

SUPRASEGMENTALS

ˈ Primary stress	ˌfoʊnəˈtɪʃən
ˌ Secondary stress	
ː Long	eː
ˑ Half long	eˑ
̆ Extra short	ĕ
. Syllable break	ɹi.ækt
| Minor (foot) group	
‖ Major (intonation) group	
‿ Linking (absence of a break)	

TONES AND WORD ACCENTS

LEVEL TONES

̋ or ˥	Extra high
́ or ˦	High
̄ or ˧	Mid
̀ or ˨	Low
̏ or ˩	Extra low

CONTOUR TONES

̌ or ˩˥	Rise
̂ or ˥˩	Fall
᷄	high rise
᷅	low rise
᷈	rise fall
↓	Downstep
↑	Upstep
etc.	

Extensions to the IPA

1.	**Other segmental features: symbols and diacritics**		
1.1.	*Place of articulation and/or co-occurring articulatory features*		
1.1.1.	[̪]	Labiodental plosives and nasal *upper teeth to lower lip*	p̪ b̪ m̪
1.1.2.	[͆]	Dentolabial plosives and nasal *lower teeth to upper lip*	p͆ b͆ m͆
1.1.3.	[͍]	Labial spreading	s͍ t͍
1.1.4.	[̪͆]	Interdental articulation *tongue tip/blade between teeth*	l̪͆ θ̪͆ l̪͆
1.1.5.	[̪͆]	Bidental articulation *teeth approximated*	h̪͆ u̪͆
1.1.6.	[̤̈]	Bidental percussive *teeth brought percussively together*	
1.2.	*Manner of articulation*		
1.2.1.	[͊]	Denasal	m͊ n͊
1.2.2.	[͋]	Nasal escape *Note*: This situation arises when an oral obstruent is intended but, because of velopharyngeal port (VPP) incompetence, audible nasal air flow results. Note that the diacritic for normal nasality refers to the presence of nasal resonance, not flow.	p͋ f͋
1.2.3.	[h͟m] [h͟n]	Nareal fricatives *Note*: These segments arise (for example) when nasal consonants are intended, but, (presumably) because of VPP incompetence, audible friction arises in the nares.	
1.2.4.	[ʩ]	Velopharyngeal fricative	
1.2.5.	[͌]	Velopharyngeal friction accompanying another sound *Note*: 1.2.4 and 1.2.5 refer to the so-called 'nasal snort', in which (usually loud) friction results from leakage through a tense, but incompletely occluded, VPP. The source of the acoustic signal is thus the VPP itself, rather than the nares.	p͌ s͌
1.2.6.	[͈] [͉]	Stronger and weaker articulation, respectively *Note*: This refers to physiological, not phonological force of articulation.	f͈ m͉
1.2.7.	[\ \ \]	Reiterated articulation *Note*: as in stuttered speech.	p\p\p
1.2.8.	[ʪ] [ʫ]	Lateralized [s] and [z], respectively *Note*: The air stream is released both centrally and laterally. The resulting fricatives are *not* the same as ɬ and ɮ.	
1.2.9.	[↑]	Whistled articulation	s↑
1.3.	*Air stream*		
1.3.1.	[↓]	Ingressive air flow for a segment which is normally egressive	p↓

N.B. X = any IPA symbol; examples of use of diacritics on IPA symbols follow explanations.

1.3.2.	[↑]	Egressive air flow for a segment which is normally ingressive *Note*: The large upwards and downwards pointing arrows may be used to indicate exhalation and inhalation, respectively.	!↑
1.3.3.	[(X)]	Silent articulation or 'mouthing'	(ʃ)
1.4.	*Vocal fold activity*		
1.4.1.	$[_{\text{v}}\ ]$ $[\ _{\text{v}}]$	Pre- and post-voicing of segments Voicing starts earlier and/or continues longer than the norm for the segment in question.	$_{\text{v}}b$ z_{v}
1.4.2.	$[\ ]_{(o)}$	Partial devoicing of a normally voiced segment	$z_{(o)}$
1.4.3.	$[\ ]_{(o}$ $[\ ]_{o)}$	Initial/final partial devoicing	$a_{(o}$ $m_{o)}$
1.4.4.	$[\ ]_{(v)}$	Partial voicing of a normally unvoiced segment	$f_{(v)}$
1.4.5.	$[\ ]_{(v}$ $[\ ]_{v)}$	Initial and final partial voicing	$h_{(v}$ $s_{v)}$
1.4.6.	[ʰ]	Pre-aspiration	ʰp

2. Degrees of indeterminancy

This is intended for those cases where, for reasons of severe distortion (e.g. due to pathological condition), the phonetic specification of an utterance cannot be made with a reasonable degree of accuracy.

2.1.	( )	A segment is perceived but no features can be identified.
	◯	The circle or balloon is the cursive form.
2.2.	(C) or (V)	Segments perceived to be consonantal or vocalic but no additional features can be identified with certainty.
2.3.	(F)	F represents an unambiguous notation for some feature of a segment that can be identified with reasonable accuracy, e.g.:
	(S) (Pal)	Stop Palatal } With no other features specifiable
2.4.	(F1, F2)	F1 and F2 represent unambiguous notations for two features of an otherwise unspecifiable segment, e.g.:
	(F, Bil)	A bilabial fricative *Note*: the comma may be omitted provided no ambiguity results.
	$(\underset{\text{v}}{S})$	Using the conventional voicing diacritic to indicate an otherwise unspecified voiced stop.
2.5.	(X)	X represents an IPA symbol used when the segment sounds like an X, but the transcriber is not quite sure, e.g.:
	(t)	What is thought to be a voiceless alveolar plosive.
2.6.	((X))	Double parentheses around one or more segments indicate that sounds were obscured by extraneous noise, e.g.: [xxxx ((2 sylls)) xxxx] *Note*: Within the double parentheses may be an indication of the number of syllables, an attempt at an orthographic or a segmental transcription, or the space may be left blank.
2.7.		The asterisk is used to make reference to segments for which no symbol is provided, e.g.: [hi hæ*], i.e. 'he has'. There should be a note elsewhere describing the way in which the segment indicated by the asterisk was produced.

3.   Voice quality

Single segments or strings of segments may be produced with a particular type of vocal cord vibration and/or supraglottal articulatory configuration. This results in secondary articulation of individual segments or an overall voice quality characterized by long-term articulatory settings.

3.1.   *Suprasegmental phonatory and articulatory features*

3.1.1.   Phonatory features.
Longer-term phonatory features that serve to characterize the speaker can be abstracted from segmental transcription by means of labelled braces, e.g.:

[xxxx {V̤ xxxxx V̤} xxxx]

for part of an utterance produced with breathy voice on all susceptible segments. The conventions for indicating long-term phonatory settings are:

V̤	breathy/whispery	V!!	ventricular/harsh
V̥	whisper	F	falsetto
V̰	creak		

3.1.2.   Articulatory features.
Longer-term articulatory features that serve to characterize the speaker can be abstracted from segmental transcription by means of labelled braces, e.g.:

[xxxx {Vʷ xxxx Vʷ} xxxx]

for part of an utterance produced with labialized articulatory setting on all susceptible segments.
Note: all IPA diacritics may be used in conjunction with V. In addition, diacritics may be used to indicate further long-term features, such as [ʹ], which may be used to indicate labiodentalized speech.

3.2   *Segmental phonatory and articulatory features*

The same diacritics used for suprasegmental voice quality and articulatory features may be used for the appropriate features of individual segments. They would be used in the same manner as all IPA diacritics.

4.   Other features of connected speech

4.1.   *Pausing*

Periods within parentheses may be used to represent pause length:

[x (.) x]   short pause
[x (..) x]   medium-length pause
[x (...) x]   long pause

4.2.   *Loudness and rate of speech*

Using conventions outlined under 3.1.

4.2.1.   Overall relative dynamic level for a number of segments:

[xxx {ᶠ xxx ᶠ} xxx]   loud speech
[xxx {ᶠᶠ xxx ᶠᶠ} xxx]   louder speech
[xxx {ₚ xxx ₚ} xxx]   quiet speech

4.2.2.   Overall relative speed of speech for a number of segments:

[xxx {allegro XXX allegro} xxx]   fast speech
[xxx {lento XXX lento} xxx]   slow speech

Chapter 3

SEGMENTAL PHONOLOGY

Introduction

As we noted in Chapter 1, one of the concerns of a phonological analysis can be to investigate the phonemes of a language, sorting out how many there are and what allophones make them up. In looking at disordered speech, many researchers have found that a phonemic approach can be useful. We can look at the output of the patient and compare it with that of the adult target, and see whether the patient has the same number of phonemes, and whether they consist of the same range of allophones. Where the two systems do not match, we can see whether the patient lacks a particular phoneme, and if so what is used in its place.

Such an approach is based on an error analysis, and within a phonemic analysis of disordered speech there has been developed a categorization of such errors. They have often been classed as "distortions" (a phonetic realization different from the target, but not so different as to be interpreted as a different phoneme), "substitutions" (a realization that is interpreted as a different phoneme, or as a sound totally outside the expected system for the language), "omission" (where no sound is attempted), and "addition" (where an extra sound is inserted in a particular example). However, this has often been felt to be a problematic classification, because it is not always clear whether a substituted sound should count as a phonetic distortion, or a phonemic substitution. Further, there have been moves away from a purely error analysis approach, to one that looks also at the system of the patient: its phonological units and their allophones, its internal consistency as well as its relation to the adult target.

Phoneme approaches are not the only way to look at phonology, and indeed in recent times have become less favoured than approaches that look for overall patterns of relationship between parts of the sound system of a language, using units smaller than phonemes or allophones. Distinctive Feature Theory sees all sounds as being made up of bundles of features, and this sort of approach is often especially useful when we examine disordered phonology. Most often, it is not an entire phoneme that has been substituted, but just an aspect of that phoneme. So, for example, if we see a change from /z/ to [s], then the feature of voicing has changed from + to -, not the entire sound. Likewise, a change from /s/ to [t] has a change in the feature continuant, or fricative. We do not have the space here to go into distinctive feature theory in detail, but those interested are recommended to refer to Clark and Yallop (1990).

A third way of examining phonological relations that has proved popular in clinical linguistics builds on both the previous approaches. This has been termed "phonological process analysis", and is a way of finding patterns of feature changes in both normal and disordered phonology. To demonstrate this approach, we can look again at our previous examples. If we see a change not only of /z/ to [s], but also /v/ → [f], /ð/ → [θ], and /ʒ/ → [ʃ], then each of these sounds has undergone the same feature change of [+voice] → [-voice]. We can then term this a general phonological process: one of fricative devoicing. Indeed, if this same change was seen affecting voiced stops converting them to voiceless stops, we would have a general process of devoicing. Taking our other example, if the change /s/ → [t] is repeated with /f/ → [p], /v/ → [b], /θ/ → [t], /ð/ → [d], /z/ → [d] etc, then we have a general process of fricative stopping (i.e. fricatives becoming stops). Many other common processes have been identified as occurring naturally during phonological acquisition, and these often seem to occur in data from phonologically delayed children. Therefore, it is claimed not only that phonological processes are an economical way of analysing data in disordered phonology, but can also have explanatory power and so can be used as a guide to remediation: following the path of normal acquisition.

Finally, we need to remember that phonology is not simply to do with single phonological units (system), but also with how these units combine (structure). Phonotactics deals with how the phonological units of a language combine to make words. For example, in English, we can have up to three consonants in a word-initial cluster, and four in word-final ones. It is often found that consonant clusters cause problems in phonologically disordered patients, so we have to be aware of cluster simplification processes of different types, and how to classify them.

Phonological disorders were for a long time the focus of most interest in speech pathology. It is not surprising, therefore, that the great majority of assessment procedures have been in this area. In terms of profiles, there are two major recent comprehensive profiles: PROPH and PACS. There are many other similar techniques, mostly not as comprehensive or recent as these. We will look at PROPH and PACS in the next two sections, and return to look at some of the others later.

3.1 PROPH

Unlike PROP and LARSP, Crystal's (1982) segmental phonological profile PROPH does not contain a developmental metric, but instead is in effect a bundle of different profiles. Below we will give an outline account of the procedure, but due its very breadth it is necessary to consult Crystal (1982) for the full details of administering PROPH.

The first page of the chart (the PROPH chart is reproduced at the end of this section) contains space at the top for the usual information on the patient and the sample. In the case of the sample, we have an added category: that of accent conventions. As noted below in Chapter 8, it is important that features of a local accent (such as /h/-dropping) are not counted as errors; therefore therapists can use this line to note down major accent features of the patient's linguistic background.

The bulk of the remainder of this first page is given over to the recording in phonetic transcription of the words of the sample. Most of these will be entered onto the grid numbered 1-100. The sample itself is recommended to be of the same type as for other profiles: interaction between patient and therapist, and spontaneous speech. However, output from picture elicitation tests could also be used. Each different word is written in ordinary orthography next to the number, and the transcription entered in the space to the right. If the word occurs more than once in the sample with the same pronunciation, then the total number of such pronunciations is added after the transcription. If the same word occurs with differing pronunciations, then alternate transcriptions are given on the transcription line, with the relevant number of times these occurred noted next to them. Words that occur very frequently (for example common grammatical words) are listed in the unnumbered box at the top: these forms are usually not entered into the subsequent analyses, but can of course be referred to if necessary.

Following on from the main transcription grid, there is a box for recording problem cases: such as where the target is difficult to guess, or the transcription was difficult to do. At the bottom of this page there is a summary section, allowing the analyst to note the total number of different words profiled as a ratio of the overall total, and to list the number of words left unanalysed due to problems.

Following this page is what Crystal (1982) calls the main part of the procedure. This is a two-page chart covering the phonological units of the English sound system, and the main consonant clusters. The groupings are based on the syllable (rather than the word), and are divided into syllable-initial (C-, CC-, CCC-), syllable-final (-C, -CC, -CCC(C)), vowels (V), syllable medial (for those examples where it is unclear from the phonetic make-up of the word whether the consonants in question belong to the first or the second syllable) (-C-, -CC(C)-), stress, and features (such as linking-r) occurring between words (Conn). Each of the consonant boxes is divided vertically between voiceless and voiced sounds, and horizontally between plosives, affricates, fricatives, nasals, and approximants. The vowel box, too, is organised into front vs. back vowels, high vs. low vowels, and monophthongs vs. diphthongs; it also contains a section for those function words (such as *a*) which consist solely of a vowel.

For the consonants and vowels, each entry consists of an overall box divided into six parts; three above a horizontal dividing line, and three below. When the sound or cluster concerned occurs in a stressed syllable, then the entries are made in the top boxes, when in unstressed syllables they are made in the lower ones. The three vertical divisions are from left-to-right, correct, omitted, and distorted/substituted. In the case of the first two, it is only necessary to note the number of occasions the sound(s) was correct or deleted, for the the final category the symbol(s) for the substituted sound(s) are entered into the box, with the number of each substitution next to it.

As might be expected, this main profiling chart can be difficult to read, as it is likely to contain a mass of information. To aid clarity, therefore, Crystal has added three supplementary pages, that therapists can use if they so wish (or use parts of). On these three pages is contained four main types of information: a phone inventory (that is, a list of the phonetic units used by the patient in the sample), a classification of these phones in terms of the adult target phones, a phonological feature and process analysis, and a section for any further analyses the therapist may wish to make.

The inventory has charts for consonants and consonant clusters (arranged by place and manner), and a vowel diagram for vowels, and boxes to show totals in the various categories. The inventory counts all phones used by the patient, whether correctly used or not, whether part of the adult target inventory or not. This section is clearly to be used as an at-a-glance account of the phonetic abilities of the patient, without regard to correctness. If we want to know how accurate the patient is as regards adult target norms, we can look at the target analysis. This also is divided into consonants, clusters and vowels, with each category dealt with in a similar, but not identical, way. We can illustrate this with the single consonant system: place and manner features are analysed separately, and correct, omitted, and substituted instances are listed in the left-hand grid. The precise nature of the errors is than entered onto the right-hand grid showing what feature was substituted for the correct one.

The feature analysis provides several matrices, the first of which is labelled (concentrating on the feature [voice]). Other features can be labelled by the analyst, and several blank matrices are left for this purpose. For the voicing feature, a place and a manner consonant matrix is provided, and the analyst notes alongside each place and each manner feature whether the [±voice] feature is maintained or lost. A similar grid is provided for consonant clusters.

The process analysis section is very simplified, with a set of process types (divided into syllable structure, assimilations, and substitutions) being listed, against which the analyst can note occurrences simply by recording the items off the preliminary grid which show these features. Unlike other profiles, PROPH does not give the phonological process a leading role in the analysis of the patient's phonology.

The final section allows the therapist to note a set of other useful features, including functional load, contrastivity (i.e. examples where a phonemeic contrast is totally maintained or totally lost), and indeterminacy (i.e. consistent problems in finding an adequate transcription).

PROPH has many advantages over other profiles, in that it has a variety of approaches from which the therapist can chose, and deals with vowels as well as consonants. However, it is still strongly biased towards a segment-by-segment approach, and might be criticised for the minimal use of processes which, whatever the argument about their psycholinguistic status, have proved useful in the analysis of disordered phonology.

3.2 PACS

Grunwell's (1985) Phonological Analysis of Child Speech (PACS) shares in many respects a common approach to that of PROPH. By this, we mean that they both use as input a sample of the patient's natural speech, and they both utilize sets of different analyses to investigate these data.

However, there is a major difference of scale between the two profiles, in that PACS consists of over a dozen different profile charts; and in terms of assessment goals. While PROPH uses what are basically phonological metrics (the patient's own system and its relationship to the target system), PACS explicitly adds in developmental and communicative adequacy measures.

Phonological Profile (PROPH)

Name _____

Age _____ Sample date _____

Duration _____

Type _____

Accent conventions _____

Gloss	Transcriptions	Gloss	Transcriptions

Gloss	Transcriptions	Gloss	Transcriptions	Gloss	Transcriptions
1		41		81	
2		42		82	
3		43		83	
4		44		84	
5		45		85	
6		46		86	
7		47		87	
8		48		88	
9		49		89	
10		50		90	
11		51		91	
12		52		92	
13		53		93	
14		54		94	
15		55		95	
16		56		96	
17		57		97	
18		58		98	
19		59		99	
20		60		100	
21		61			
22		62		Problems	
23		63			
24		64			
25		65			
26		66			
27		67			
28		68			
29		69			
30		70			
31		71			
32		72			
33		73			
34		74			
35		75			
36		76			
37		77			
38		78			
39		79			
40		80			

Total word types		TTR	
Total word tokens		Total problems	
Repeated forms		Total unintelligible	
Variant forms		Analysed:unanalysed	

29

The Clinician's Guide to Linguistic Profiling

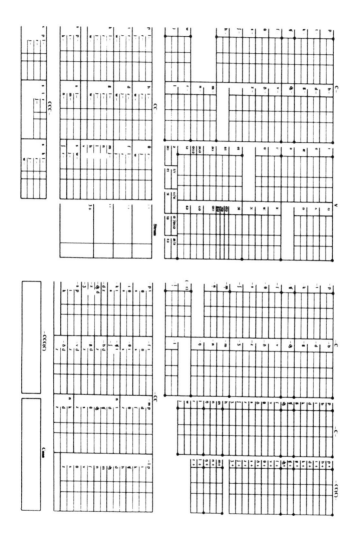

30

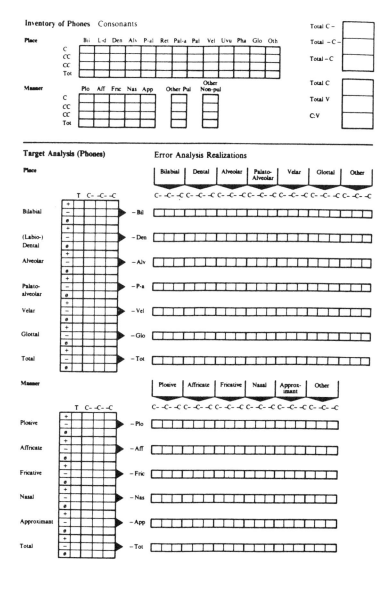

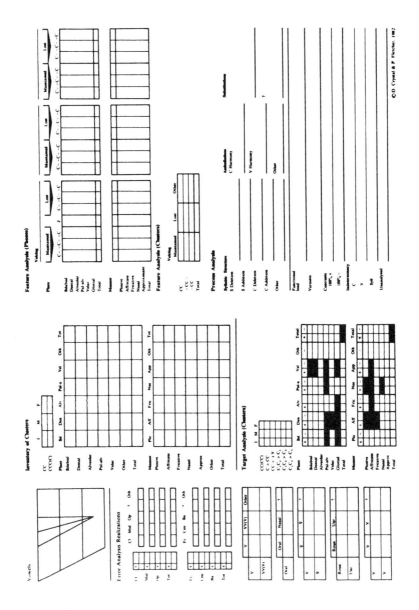

Due to the potential length of the PACS procedure, we have not included all the charts provided in Grunwell (1985); however, as the author points out, the core of the profile is smaller (with optional components available to the clinician for specific aspects of the child's phonology), and examples of the use of these core charts (from Grunwell, 1988) are given at the end of this section.

Grunwell (1988, p225) notes that PACS is capable of meeting the requirements of an adequate phonological profile, in that the analyses include the following:

1. analysis of the phonetic range and distribution of consonant sounds occurring in the child's spoken language, that is the *phonetic inventory*.

2. analysis of the child's use of this phonetic inventory at different positions in word and syllable structure, and the combinations of consonants that occur at these structural positions, that is the *contrastive system* and the *phonotactic inventory*.

In order to meet these aims, there are (amongst the profile charts) specific charts dealing with the child's phonetic and phonological system and how it relates to the adult target system (charts 1-4 at the end of this section); and charts dealing with a developmental assessment of the phonological processes evident in the data (charts 5-7 at the end of this section).

Further charts exist dealing with a distinctive feature analysis, assessment of loss of phonemic contrasts, assessment of variability, and assessment of homophony. To some extent, these are expansions of features occurring at the end of the PROPH chart, but they also highlight the concern of PACS to provide an analysis of communicative adequacy. Readers interested in these areas are referred to Grunwell (1985) for a description of these charts and how to use them.

The initial stages of PACS require the transcription of the sample into narrow phonetic symbolization, and the entry of the transcription onto the initial chart. This is laid out in a similar way to PROPH, but does not have a box for common words. It does, however, have space for the phonemic transcription of the adult target for each entry, and room for connected speech data. The phoneme realisation chart also bears similarities to PROPH's segment classification chart. In PACS, the phonemes are listed in four columns corresponding to the four places in syllable structure (see below) rather than the three of PROPH, and while the three box layout (correct, zero, incorrect) is retained, there is no differentiation between stressed and unstressed occurrences.

The two main differences between the PROPH and PACS approaches at this initial stage, however, are firstly that vowels are excluded - PACS is solely concerned with consonants. This has to be regretted as a retrograde step, particularly in light of the recent work on vowels in disordered phonology (see Stoel-Gammon and Beckett Herrington, 1990, Pollock and Keiser, 1990, and Pollock and Hall, 1991).

Secondly, Grunwell is firm on the exclusion of a word-medial category. PACS requires that four word positions are recognized: syllable initial, word initial (SIWI), syllable initial within word (SIWW), syllable final within word (SFWW), and syllable final, word final (SFWF). While Crystal (1982) argued that it was not always easy to locate syllable boundaries in word-medial position (see his examples in Crystal, 1982, p63), Grunwell (1985) requires that this be done, and provides guidelines on segmentation (see p11). Needless to say, while these guidelines are relatively straightforward, they will not always coincide with every speaker's intuitions, and not all phonologists will agree on them (see for example, Jassem's 1990 discussion of this topic).

To illustrate the application of the core charts of PACS, we will follow Grunwell (1988) and give a brief description of the charts included at the end of this section. The first of these contains the patient's phonetic inventory and phonetic distribution. This analysis enables the clinician to analyse the patient's phonetic capabilities without regard to the target realizations or to the phonological (i.e. contrastive) use these phones may be put to. The upper table arranges the patient's phones in terms of place and manner labels, while the lower table shows where in the word structure these phones occur (SIWI, SIWW, SFWW, SFWF) in singletons and in clusters. As can be seen from the example, numbers can be used to mark rare occurrences. This chart provides ready access to the patient's overall phonetic capabilities, and sounds missing in comparison with the target system, or additional sounds, can easily be spotted.

The second chart continues the analysis of the child's system, but introduces explicit contrasts with the adult target system. The clinician needs to work out the contrastive phones (i.e. phonological units) used by the child to signal differences of meaning. These are then plotted onto the relevant grid (according to position in word structure) to show the direct relationship between the child's form and the adult form. The grids used here are one of the novel features of Grunwell's work, and provide an easily understood contrastive analysis.

The next two charts provide in-depth coverage of the phonotactic capabilities of the patient, and as Grunwell notes, this is an area often ignored by other procedures. The first chart shows a wide range of phonotactic possibilities in monosyllables, disyllables (of two different stress patterns), and polysyllables. The grids are used to enumerate the different ways in which the patient realised adult target word structures. The second chart allows the clinician to summarize this information, and to show what phones the child used for certain common adult target consonant clusters. Grunwell (1988) notes that it is often not necessary to conduct a phonotactic analysis, but the fact that PACS provides this possibility is a mark of its flexibility.

The remaining charts constitute the developmental metric of PACS. Charts 5 and 6 are for a phonological process analysis of quite a sophisticated kind (in comparison, for example, with PROPH). Following her own analysis of processes as set out in Grunwell (1982, 1987), the processes are divided between systemic and structural simplifications, and a wide range of processes (not just those usually identified as "natural") are included. For the precise meaning and examples of the various process types, readers are referred to Grunwell (1985). The charts allow not only for the noting of the use of each process along with examples, but also for noting the frequency of use in potential environments - clearly a guide as to whether a process is being eliminated[1] or is still active.

The final chart in our selection provides for the developmental assessment of the patient. Based on Grunwell's previous work on phonological development (e.g. 1982, 1987), the chart provides seven chronological stages from 0;9 to 4;6+ (the same stages used in LARSP, see Chapter 5). At each stage are listed both the contrastive phone system, and phonological processes found normally at that age range. As is shown in the chart, a patient's phonological stage can be worked out using this chart.

Apart from filling in the core and optional charts to gain a profile of a patient's phonological capabilities, users of PACS can also attempt evaluations of the patterns found. Grunwell (1988) points out that terms such as "delayed development", "uneven development" and "deviant development" can be assigned to different patients. Data obtained from PACS can also be used to attempt explanations of different patterns of phonological disorder. It is beyond the scope of this chapter to detail these areas of analysis, but Grunwell (1988) utilizes several case studies to illustrate them.

PACS is clearly a longer procedure (potentially) than PROPH, and appears at first sight more complex. However, the multiplicity of charts acts in reality to produce a simpler step-by-step approach, and allows clincians to chose just those analysis procedures they feel most appropriate.

3.3 Other Profiles

The large number of guides to phonological assessment, together with formal systems of tests and profiles means that it is impossible in this section to do more than simply list a selection of the more popular of these with a brief description. We exclude those procedures that are clearly tests (of a similar type to the articulation tests described in Chapter 2). Many procedures are linked closely to one particular approach to phonology, and we will list these other profiles according to which approach they espouse. Computerized profiles are described in Pye (1987), Pye and Ingram (1988), Long and Fey (1990a) and Shriberg (1986).

Phonetic Inventory

© Pamela Grunwell, 1985.
Published by
The NFER-NELSON Publishing Company Ltd.,
Darville House, 2 Oxford Road East, Windsor,
Berkshire SL4 1DF.

Name ....Simon....4;7.........

	Labial	Dental	Alveolar	Post-Alveolar	Palatal	Velar	Glottal	Other
Nasal	m		n					
Plosive	p b		t d				ʔ	
Fricative								
Affricate								
Approximant	w		l		j			
Other								

Marginal Phones: t ʊ

Phonetic Distribution

	Single Consonants					Consonant Clusters			
	SIWI	SIWW	SFWW	SFWF		SIWI	SIWW	SFWW	SFWF
Nasal	m n	m n	m¹ n	m n					mpt¹ nt¹
Plosive	p¹ b t² d	p² b¹ ʔ d	ʔ	p b¹ t d ʔ					pt¹
Fricative									
Affricate									
Approximant	w l j	w l		t ʊ					
Other									

Systems of Contrastive Phones and Contrastive Assessments

PACS © Pamela Grunwell, 1985.

Published by
The NFER–NELSON Publishing Company Ltd.,
Darville House, 2 Oxford Road East, Windsor,
Berkshire SL4 1DF.

Name .... $Simon$ ... $(4;7)$ ....

Syllable Initial Word Initial

m		n							
m		n							
p b	b b	t d	d d	tʃ d	dʒ d	k d	g d		
f w	v w	θ j / s j	ð /// / z ///	ʃ j					
w w	r w / l l	j j	L	h ///					

Syllable Initial Within Word

m		n						
m		n						
p p	b b	t d ?	d d	tʃ d	dʒ d	k ?	g d	
f w	v b	θ /// / s ?h	ð d / z d	ʃ ///	ʒ ///			
w w	r w / l l	j j	h ///					

Syllable Final Word Final

m		n					ŋ	n
m		n					ŋ	n
p p	b b	t t	d d	tʃ t	dʒ d	k ?ø	g d	
f ø	v d	θ ø / s ø	ð /// / z d	ʃ ø	ʒ ///			
r /// / l l								

Phonotactic Possibilities:
Contrastive Analysis

PACS

© Pamela Grunwell, 1985.
Published by
The NFER-NELSON Publishing Company Ltd.,
Darville House, 2 Oxford Road East, Windsor,
Berkshire SL4 1DF

Name .... Simon 4;7

Child

Monosyllables	V	CV	VC	CVC	CCV	VCC	CCVC	CCVCC	CCCVCC	CCCV	CCCVC	CCCVCC	CVSC CVC							
V																				
CV	1												1							
VC																				
CVC	9	28											33							
CCV	3												3							
VCC																				
CCVC	1	15											16							
CVCC	1	1											2							
CCVCC				1									1							
CCCVCC					1					1			1							
CCCV																				
CCCVC																				
CCCVCC												1	1							
CVVk																				
	15	43		2						11	11	68								

Child

Disyllables ' ᴗ	VCV	CVCV	VCVC	CVCVC	VC.CV	CVC.CV	VC.CVC	CVCVC	CCVCV	CVC.CVC	CV.CCV	CVC.CVC	CCV.CCV	CCV.CCV	CVC.CCVC	CVCVCC	CVC.CVC	CVC.CVC	CCVC.CVCC		CVCV ' CV
VCV																					
CVCV	7																		7		
VCVC																					
CVCVC			5																5		
VC.CV																					
CVC.CV				1															1	1	
VC.CVC																					
CVC.CVC																					
CCVCV	1																		1		
CCVCVC			2																3		
CCV.CVC				1															1		
CV.CCV																					
CVC.CCV																					
CVC.CCVC																					
CCV.CCV																					
CCV.CCVC																					
CCVCC																					
CVCVCC																					
CCVCVCC																					
CCVC.CVCC																					
CCVkCCVC			1																1		
CCVC.CV				1																	
	16	13	2	1								(19)		20	1						

Child

Disyllables ᴗ '						

Polysyllabic Targets	Child's Realizations	No. Tokens
'VCV,CCVC	VCV,CVC	1
'CVCV CCVC	'CVCV,CVC	1
'CVC, CVCVC	'CVC, CVCV	1

Phonotactic Analysis:
Contrastive Assessment

PACS

© Pamela Grunwell, 1985.
Published by
The NFER-NELSON Publishing Company Ltd.,
Darville House, 2 Oxford Road East, Windsor,
Berkshire SL4 1DF.

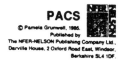

Name ....S.i.m.o.n...4.;.7.............

Phonotactic Potential

Word Structure	No.	No. Att.	Phonotactic Possibilities	Attempted Target Structures	Child's Canonical Structure	No.	No. Att.
Monosyllable	62	62	$C_1 V C_{0-3}$	$C_{1-3} V C_{0-3}$	C V	15	1
					C VC	43	35
Disyllable	19	20	$CVC_1 C_1 V C_{0-1}$	CVCC VC $_{1-3\ 0-1\ 1-2\ 0-1}$	'CVCV	8	7
					'CVCVC	8	5
Polysyllable	4	3	VCV, CVC CVCVCV CVCV, CVC CVC, CVCV	VCV, CCVC (CVC,CV) CVCV, CCVC CVC, CVCVC	—		—

Contrastive Assessment of Clusters: Summary

Syllable Initial Word Initial

Child Realization		Target
m		s m
n		s n
b		s p
d		s t
		s k
b		p r
b		p l
b		b r
b		b l
	w	t r
	w	d r
	w	k w
	w	k r
d		k l
	w	g r
d		g l
		f r
w		f l
	w	θ r
	w	s w
	ʟ	s l
		ʃ r
		s p r
		s p l
		s t r
		s k w
		s k r

Syllable Final Word Final

C₁	C₂	C₃	Target C, +
m	p	t	m pʃ
n	t		n t
			ŋ
p	t		pʃ
			b
			t
			d
			tʃ
∅	t		dʒ
			ks
			g
			f
			v
			θ
			ð
			s
			z
			ʃ
			ʒ
			l

Phonological Process Analysis: Systemic Simplifications

PACS

© Pamela Grunwell, 1985.
Published by
The NFER-NELSON Publishing Company Ltd.,
Darville House, 2 Oxford Road East, Windsor,
Berkshire SL4 1DF.

Name .... Simon h.7 ....

Phonological Process		Tokens No./No. Poss.	Details and Examples	Other Realizations	Notes
FRONTING	velars	25/38		WW; WF /k/ → [ʔ] or ∅; and ∅ in clusters	
	palato-alveolars	13/17	/tʃ/ → [t; d] /dʒ/ → [d]	/ʃ/ → [j] SIWI → ∅ SFWF	
STOPPING	/f/	0/9		Gliding SI ∅ SFWF	
	/v/	3/4	SFWF → [d]	Gliding SIWI	
	/θ/	0/4		Gliding SIWI ∅ in clusters; SFWF	
	/ð/	1/1	SIWW → [d]		
	/s/	3/20	SFWF clusters → [t]	Gliding SIWI ∅ in clusters; SFWF	
	/z/	6/7	SIWW SFWF } → [d]	SFWF → ∅	
	/ʃ/	0/4		Gliding SIWI ∅ SFWF	
	/tʃ/	6/6	SIWI and SFWF → [t d]		
	/dʒ/	7/7	SIWI, SIWW and SFWF → [d]		
	/l/	0/16			See below
	/r/	0/19			See Gliding
GLIDING	/r/	16/19	SIWI and clusters and SIWW → [w]	Deleted in clusters with LABIAL plosives	
	/l/	0/16			Realised correctly
	fricatives	15/50	/f v/ → [w] } SIWI /θ s/ → [j]	SFWF see Stopping	Only occurs SIWI
CSV	WI and WF				
	Voicing WI	19	/p t k tʃ/ SIWI	Gliding of Forbs Fricatives involves Voicing	
	Voicing WW	2			
	Devoicing WF				
GLOTTAL REPLACEMENT	WI				
	WW	4	/t k/ SIWW; /k/ SFWW		
	WF	4	/k/ only		
GLOTTAL INSERTION					

Phonological Process Analysis:
Structural Simplifications

PACS

© Pamela Grunwell, 1985.
Published by
The NFER-NELSON Publishing Company Ltd.,
Darville House, 2 Oxford Road East, Windsor,
Berkshire SL4 1DF.

Name .... SiMON 4:7 ....

Phonological Process	Tokens No./No. Poss.	Details and Examples	Other Realizations	Notes
W.S.D. pretonic	0/0			
posttonic	0/23			
F.C.D. nasals	0/16			
plosives	3/24	/k/ only	/k/ also realised as [ʔ]	
fricatives	8/16	/f s ʃ/	Lenis fricatives stopped	Only fortis fricatives deleted
affricatives	0/6		Affricates stopped.	
clusters −1	1/5	/ks/ → [t]	Other clusters realised	NB Singleton /k/
−2+	1/5	/ks/ → [ø]	as clusters	and fortis fricatives deleted
VOCALIZATION /l/				Vocalic lateral /l/ acceptable
other C				
REDUPLICATION complete				⎫ Not
partial				⎭ evidenced
CONSONANT HARMONY velar				⎫
alveolar				⎪
labial				⎬ Not evidenced
manner				⎪
other				⎭
S.I. CLUSTER REDUCTION plosive + approx.	15/15	LAB/VEL}+/l/ → STOP PL/VEL}+/r/ → [w]		Normal and unusual patterns
fricative + approx.	5/5	/fl/ → [w] ie fric. /θr/ → [w] ie /r/		Normal and unusual patterns
/s/ + plosive	4/4	/s/ deleted; plosive retained		Normal pattern
/s/ + nasal	2/2	Nasal retained		Normal pattern
/s/ + approx.	3/3	Approx. retained		Possible normal pattern
/s/ + plosive + approx.	2/2	Approx. retained		Unusual pattern

Developmental Assessment

PACS
© Pamela Grunwell, 1985.
Published by
The NFER-NELSON Publishing Company Ltd.,
Darville House, 2 Oxford Road East, Windsor.
Berkshire SL4 1DF.

Name ...... Simon 4.7 ......

		Labial	Lingual	Protowords and First Words:
Stage I (0;9 – 1;6)	Nasal			Show phonetic variability and all phon processes. *Examples*
	Plosive			
	Fricative			
	Approximant			

Stage II (1;6 – 2;0)	m		n			Reduplication	FRONTING ✱	✓
	p b	t	d			Consonant Harmony	STOPPING	
						FINAL CONS. DELETION	GLIDING	
	w					CLUSTER REDUCTION	C.S.VOICING	
							✱ always operates	

Stage III (2;0 – 2;6)	(m)		(n)		(ŋ)		Fronting /long.fircs wf	✓
	(p)(b)	(t)	(d)		(d)(g)✗	Final Cons. Deletion ✱ ✓	STOPPING — affrics.	✓
						CLUSTER REDUCTION ✓	GLIDING	✓
	(w)	(l)	(j)		(h)	✱ fortis frics. only	C.S.VOICING – SIWI	
							GLIDING of FRICS	

Stage IV (2;6 – 3;0)	m		n		ŋ		STOPPING/v ð z tʃ dʒ/	
	p b	t	d		k g	Final Cons. Deletion	FRONTING/ʃ/ →[s]	
	f	s				CLUSTER REDUCTION	GLIDING	
	w	(l)		j	h		C.S.Voicing	

Stage V (3;0 – 3;6)	m		n		ŋ		STOPPING/v ð z/	
	p b	t	d	(tʃ)	k g	Clusters used:	FRONTING/ʃ tʃ dʒ/	
	f	s		(ʃ)		obs. + approx.	GLIDING	
	w	l		j	h	/s/ + cons.	/θ/ →[f]	

Stage VI (3;6 – 4;6)	m		n		ŋ		/ð/ →[d] or [v]	
	p b	t	d	tʃ dʒ	k g	Clusters used:	PALATALIZATION/ʃ tʃ dʒ/	
	f v	s	z ʃ			obs + approx.	GLIDING	
	w	l	(r)	j	h	/s/ + cons	/θ/ →[f]	

Stage VII (4;6 <)	m		n		ŋ		/ð/ →[d] or [v]	
	p b	t	d	tʃ dʒ	k g	Clusters used:	/r/ →[w] or [ʋ]	
	f v	θ s ð z	ʃ (ʒ)			obs + approx.	/θ/ →[f]	
	w	l	r	j	h	/s/ + cons.		

Comments and Notes

Velars are absent from Simon's system.
but approximant subsystem more developed
than at a normal Stage II.
Gliding of fricatives is an unusual early process.

Approaches that rely mainly on producing a description of the patient's disordered phonology as a system in its own right, and then a contrastive analysis with the adult target, include Stoel-Gammon and Dunn's (1985) "independent analysis", and "relational analysis" (though this latter also comes under the natural processes approach). Similarly, Elbert and Gierut's (1986) "assessing productive phonological knowledge" procedure requires an independent analysis of the disordered system, though Grunwell (1987) criticizes the way the contrastive assessment aspect of their procedure operates.

Distinctive feature and generative phonological approaches to assessment have not, on the whole, proved popular or successful. We might mention here McReynolds and Engmann's (1976) "distinctive feature analysis of misarticulations" and Compton and Hutton's (1978) "Compton-Hutton phonological assessment". However, both of these can be criticized (see Grunwell, 1987) as not providing an output suitable for planning remediation.

Finally, there are a number of procedures based on natural phonological processes (some with other approaches built in as well). We can note here in chronological order of publication PPA (Phonological Process Analysis, Weiner, 1979), NPA (Natural Process Analysis, Shriberg and Kwiatkowski, 1980), APP (Assessment of Phonological Processes, Hodson, 1980), and PPACL (Procedures for the Phonological Analysis of Children's Language, Ingram, 1981); however, of these, only NPA and PPACL use spontaneous rather than elicited speech as input, and we will look further at these two only.

NPA is limited in terms of the data that is included in the input (only monosyllables, only first use of a word), and in the number of processes listed on the chart. PPACL, however, contains a substitution analysis as well as a process one, allows for the measurement of frequency of occurrence of a process, and includes a range of normal and unusual processes. We might conclude, however, that PROPH and PACS offering, as they do, a range of possible analyses will be more useful than procedures concentrating on only one.

Chapter 4

SUPRASEGMENTAL PHONOLOGY

Introduction

As we have noted previously, there are several areas of the sound system of a language that are not restricted to the segment, but have "domains" that may stretch over several segments. These are often just as important to the correct transmission of an oral message as the individual sound segments themselves, so any disorder of suprasegmental phonology (often termed a "prosodic disorder") can be most disruptive and need effective treatment.

However, suprasegmental phonology has proved, by and large, more difficult to describe than segmental; with the result that, whereas numerous assessment procedures exist to deal with the latter, the former is generally not well served.

Before we go on to look in detail at one such "prosodic profile", we need to be aware of what phenomena are generally classed under the heading of suprasegmental phonology.

We can list the features most commonly classed under this heading as follows: pitch, stress, loudness, speed of speech, and voice quality. Pitch, when used linguistically (i.e. within a language for meaning purposes), is usually called "intonation"; and patterns of stress, together with loudness, speech speed, pausing etc, are often grouped together as "rhythm".

Finally, "voice quality" is a term that covers a variety of articulatory features. It can refer to the actions of the vocal folds (i.e. "whisper" and "creak" as voice qualities), or to settings of the supra-laryngeal vocal tract (such as a "palatal voice quality"). It often has attached to it impressionistic terms such as "hoarse" or "tight". We have not the space here to examine in detail the phonetic description of voice quality (or indeed any other of these suprasegmental features). Readers wishing to know more are recommended to Ball (1989).

While all of the above noted suprasegmental features can be

found disturbed in non-normal speech, it is probably true that it is pitch and voice quality that are found most often. To date, no profile of quite the type we have been examining in this book has been proposed for the analysis of voice quality. This is a notoriously difficult area to deal with, as impressionistic descriptions of different voice qualities are imprecise, and instrumental analyses difficult due to the multiplicity of factors that can be involved in the production of a particular quality (see Laver 1980). In the final part of this chapter, then, we propose a new profile of voice quality.

We find then, that the only profile currently available that actually deals with suprasegmental phonology is restricted almost entirely to pitch: i.e. intonation (Crystal, 1982).

4.1 PROP

The PROP technique is centred on a single page profile chart that is loosely developmental in its layout. It assumes an ability to transcribe a stretch of speech in both a segmental and suprasegmental manner. By this is meant that a transcription of the pitch movements of the speaker must be made, and matched to a transcription (phonetic or orthographic) of the individual speech sounds of the speaker. This is by no means an easy task, and some training is normally required; even clinicians used to segmental phonetic analysis experience difficulty in the recognition of prosodic features.

The PROP chart is divided into three main parts: *tone unit* analysis, *tone* analysis, and *tonicity* analysis. We will look at each of these terms in turn before going on to see how they are used in the profile. The chart itself is given at the end of this section.

Tone unit is the term used to describe the particular stretch of speech over which an intonation pattern operates. This stretch of speech often coincides with syntactic units (such as the clause or phrase), but in rapid speech longer stretches might be used, and in deviant speech, both longer and shorter tone units may occur that may not coincide with syntactic units.

Within each tone unit there will be one major pitch movement, termed here the *tone* (in other works, "nuclear tone/nucleus" or "tonic" may be used for this feature). This tone will be one of a small set of major tones used in the language or dialect, whose use is usually associated with particular shades of meaning (such as "certainty" or "questioning"). Crystal (1982), for PROP, recognises seven such tones (though a different seven from those classified by O'Connor and Arnold (1973)). These are as follows, using the diacritics suggested by Crystal (1982, p116):

Freda's gòing	falling (neutral; matter of fact)
Freda's góing	rising (questioning, surprised)
Freda's gōing	level (routine, bored)
Freda's gŏing	fall-rise (warning, caution)
Freda's gôing	rise-fall (definite, impressed)
Frèda's góing	fall+rise (extra emphasis on *Freda*)
Fréda's gòing	rise+fall (extra emphasis on *Freda*)

These last two are termed *compound tones*, and are grouped together on the chart, and represented by C. (It is worth noting that many researchers, such as O'Connor and Arnold (1973) recognise high and low varieties of the simple rise and the simple fall tones; which they further claim have different meaning associations.)

PROP also uses some further diacritics to mark other prosodic features that the clinician may wish to note. They include marks of syllabic stress ('$ for stressed syllable [$ = syllable]; "$ for extra stressed syllable); marks for noticeable steps up or down in pitch compared to the previous syllable: ↑ and ↓; marks for short pauses (shorter than a speaker's rhythm unit): . , and for a pause equivalent to a speaker's rhythm unit: - . They also recommend that stretches of speech with a particular voice quality should be marked with single quote marks, and the relevant description placed in the margin of the transcription (the IPA Extensions now recommend the use of braces for this purpose, see below in 4.2).

The final aspect of intonation investigated by PROP involves *tonicity*. This is the term used to describe how the nuclear tone is positioned within the tone unit. Tone units themselves may contain pitch movements before and after the nuclear tone (and of course these may need to be noted), and they may have nuclear tones placed early or late in the tone unit (assuming it is long enough for this to happen). This placement can affect the meaning portrayed by the utterance:

Fred *saw Freda yesterday* ~ *Fred saw Freda* **yesterday**

If we compare these two examples, we note that the first seems to be in response to a request about who saw Freda, or a contradiction that, for example, it was Ferdy not Fred who saw Freda. The second is supplying information about when the event took place, or contradicting a claim that it was today.

We can now turn attention to the way in which these three aspects of intonation are entered onto the PROP chart. The analysis of the tone unit is mainly syntactic: that is the tone units are analysed to see which syntactic unit they coincide with. The syntactic units recognised for this purpose are clause, phrase, word, and units above the clause (Cl+), and above the phrase but below the clause (Cl-). The number of each tone unit type is recorded onto the chart opposite the category label. Crystal (1982) illustrates these levels of analysis with the following examples:

clause:	*'when he cómes/ 'I'll be òut*
phrase:	*a 'big càt/*
word:	*yès/*
Cl+:	*I knòw he'll be hére/*
Cl-:	*'that man is/ an idiot*

The chart also allows for the marking of problematic cases. Four types are recognised: incomplete, where hesitation, false starts etc result in an unfinished intonation pattern; indeterminate, where there is any uncertainty as to whether a complete tone unit has been accomplished (for example during "overlaps", when two speakers are speaking at the same time); stereotypes, where set patterns are continually employed for a set utterance or, for example, where rhymes are recited; and imitations, where the patient is simply imitating the therapist, and we cannot know, therefore, whether the patient has active control over this pattern.

This part of the chart is also to be used for a functional analysis of the tone units. The box labelled "functions" is an attempt to provide an analysis (albeit basic) of the functions of the intonation patterns used by the patient. There are no agreed set of labels we can use in the analysis of the semantics of intonation as each researcher in the field seems to coin their own labels. Crystal therefore recommends that the therapist uses their own terms to describe those functions of the patient's intonation that appear worthy of note. These might be unusual functions (such as "uses ˇ for ˋ") or simply a list of the number of times a particular function occurs (e.g. "questioning 15").

The second part of the chart concerns the marking of nuclear tones. Space is provided for the analyst to enter the nuclear tones used in the sample (which can be numbered to aid memory). This is not a full transcription of the pitch usage of the patient, as only the nuclear tones are used, with pre- and post-nuclear patterns omitted. Beneath this transcription space is a table onto which the tone information is entered. This table is devised to contain a developmental metric, in that the various nuclear tone types are listed down the left-hand side in developmental order. Columns in this matrix allow each nuclear tone to be entered either as "normal" (∅), or as having a narrower/wider pitch range than normal (N/W), lower starting point than normal (↓), higher starting point than normal/probable higher starting point than normal (↑/?↑), or that the tone is produced with extra stress ("). As always, an "other" column is included where can be marked information concerning other features of the pitch, such as unusual voice quality.

Finally, we can look at the tonicity section. Again, there are sections to mark indeterminate, stereotypical and imitative placement of the nuclear tone within the tone unit. The matrix for marking all other aspects of tonicity is divided along three different criteria. The first is whether the placement is on the final item of the tone unit (most common in normal speech), or on any pre-final item. Secondly, a distinction is made between lexical (or contentive) and grammatical (or functive) carriers of nuclear tone. In terms of using tone to distinguish words, there are clearly more lexical words (nouns, verbs, etc) we can distinguish than grammatical (e.g. prepositions, conjunctions). Such an analysis, therefore, will aid decisions on intervention, as different strategies will be needed if problems arise with tone placement on

49

lexical words than if they occur with grammatical words.

The last distinction made in this section is between appropriate and inappropriate use of tonicity (marked here by a tick and a cross). By using all three aspects together, we get a picture of where the majority of tone placements occur, on what type of item, and whether this appears appropriate with regard to normal speakers or not. Again, as with other sections of the chart, this gives clear guidelines as to whether therapeutic intervention is required, and where it should concentrate.

Below this part of the chart is an "other" section. This allows the marking of other aspects of the pitch of the tone units apart from the nuclear tone (i.e. pre- and post-nuclear) where they are of interest; other non-pitch aspects of the tone units (such as tempo, and loudness); prosodic features that extend over longer periods of the speaker's utterances; and paralinguistic features such as voice quality. Very little space is given to these last two features, however, and patients exhibiting disorders mainly in these areas might well be profiled on the PROVOQ chart described in the next section. Long (1987) and Long and Fey (1990a) describe a computerized version of PROP.

4.2 PROVOQ

As mentioned above, there have been few attempts to provide assessment materials in suprasegmental phonology apart from the area of intonation. The area of Voice Quality, however, is an important one for speech pathology, as a variety of disorders can affect this aspect of speech. In this book we introduce a new profile for voice quality to complement PROP (though see also the recent work of Shriberg, Kwiatkowski and Rasmussen, 1989a, b)

This profile has been named PROVOQ: the PRofile Of VOice Quality. Like PROP it is a one-page profile, but lacking any kind of developmental scaling (for which there is little evidence), it works much more like a check-list, in the way of the pragmatic profiles discussed in Chapter 7. The Profile covers two other suprasegmental features other than voice quality: speech tempo, and loudness.

Prosody Profile (PROP)

Name		Duration	
Age	Sample date	Type	

Tone Unit (0; 9 +)   Total   Average words

Structures

Incomplete	Indeterminate	Stereotyped	Imitation
Clause		**Functions**	
Phrase			
Word			
Other Cl +			
Cl −			

Tone (0; 9 +)

Data Variants

Deviant

Summary: Other   N   W   ↓   ?↑   ↑   "   ∅

0; 9 +	−								
	`								
1; 0 +	´								
1; 3 +	^								
	˘								
1; 6 +	C								
	?								

Tonicity (1; 6 +)

Indeterminate   Stereotyped   Imitation

	Non Final		Final	
Simple	✓	×	✓	×
Lexical				
Grammatical				
Complex	NF + NF		NF + F	

Other

Tone unit pitch	Prosodic features (TU +)
Tone unit other	Paraling features

© David Crystal 1981

51

The Profile recognises two main ways in which non-normal voice quality may manifest itself in a speech sample: the voice quality itself may be consistent or nearly so (in that, for example, breathy voice may be used throughout the sample, or consistently through a connected part of it), or it may be intermittent (in that a specific voice quality may occur only in certain small parts of the sample, or indeed, in certain words or parts of words). To accomodate this difference, the Profile form is divided into two parts: one where the consistent voice qualities can be marked, and the amount of this usage noted as a proportion of the whole sample; and secondly, a part to note intermittent usage of non-normal voice qualities. This is done by transcribing the parts of the utterance demonstrating the voice quality into a section (as in PROP) set aside for transcriptions. (See PROVOQ Chart, included at the end of this section.)

The Profile chart contains at the top space for the usual patient information, such as name, age, sample date, sample duration and sample type. Following this is the section for consistent voice quality. Eight different voice quality categories are listed using the appropriate symbols of the Extensions to the IPA: breathy voice, whisper, creak, harsh or ventricular voice, and falsetto as aspects of phonation; and two supralaryngeal categories: V^x as a cover symbol for features such as labialized, palatalized, velarized, etc, and $\tilde{V}$ for nasalized; an "other" category is also included.

For each of these eight types a comment column is available to record more detailed information (such as degree of severity/ intelligibility, mixture of phonation types as in whispery creak, or specification of supralaryngeal type). As noted above, it is also possible to show the approximate amount of the sample that was made up of the non-normal voice quality, through symbols marking quarter, half, three-quarters and whole. For each voice quality marked, it is also possible to mark whether the speaker was using loud or soft voice (*p-f*), and slow or fast tempo (*allegro–lento*), again using the conventions of the Extensions to the IPA. These last features can also be used to profile speakers who have otherwise normal voice qualities; in this case the "other" category would be employed, glossed as "normal" in the comment column.

The section for intermittent voice qualities provides space for several lines of transcription (which if necessary can be continued on the reverse of the form). It is suggested that fragments of the sample be recorded here that contain the non-normal voice qualities; such features being marked off by braces from the rest of the utterance following the conventions of the Extensions to the IPA. This can be illustrated as follows: /aɪ wʌndə {F wen hil əraɪv F}/, which shows that just the last three words were said with a falsetto voice.

Beneath the section for transcriptions there are two summary boxes. Here can be summarized the number of each voice type included in the transcriptions, and the number of times soft/loud, or fast/slow speech styles were noted.

Clearly, patients may well present who use a specific non-normal voice quality consistently through a large, connected part of the sample, and then intermittently for the remainder. In such cases it is recommended that both parts of the chart be utilised to demonstrate the patient's change of usage pattern. It would be as well, also, to note any characteristics of the respective parts of the utterance which might account for the patient's altered strategy.

These voice-related features are not subjected to any kind of measurement (though degree of intelligibility can of course be marked in the comment column). This is because, unlike other aspects, they don't fall readily into developmental stages, and any external measure is bound to be artificial to some extent. We therefore see this Profile more as a checklist for specific patients, where will be recorded, and easily retrieved, information on what non-normal voice quality patterns a patient uses, to what extent they use them, and whether they coincide with other features of connected speech such as tempo and loudness. To this extent, PROVOQ aids in planning intervention because it shows clearly the precise areas of concern.

Profile in Voice Quality (PROVOQ)

Name _____ Duration _____

Age _____ Sample date _____ Type _____

Consistent Voice Qualities

Voice Quality	Occurence in sample				p – f	all – len	comments
V̤							
V̇							
V̱							
V!!							
F							
Vˣ							
Ṽ							
other							

Intermittent Voice Qualities

Transcriptions _____

_____

_____

_____

_____

_____

_____

_____

Summary

V̤	F
V̇	Vˣ
V̱	Ṽ
V!!	other

p – f
all – len

Chapter 5

MORPHOLOGY AND SYNTAX

Introduction

Grammatical analysis of a language deals with both word structure (morphology) and sentence structure (syntax). Before we can describe grammatical profiles for disordered language, we need to take a closer look at these two sub-components, first discussed in Chapter 1.

Morphology deals, amongst other things, with the use of affixes (prefixes and suffixes). In English, affixes can be used for two main purposes: derivational and inflectional. Derivational affixes are found when a new lexical item is constructed out of an existing one, e.g. "beauty" → "beauti+ful" → "beautiful+ly". Inflectional affixes, on the other hand, do not create a new lexical item, but express grammatical relations such as plurality (in nouns), or tense or aspect (in verbs); examples include "cat" → "cat+s", "walk" → "walk+ing", "big" → "bigg+er" → "bigg+est". (See also the discussion on morphology in Chapter 1.) By and large, whereas derivational morphology does not regularly feature as a problem in the disordered language literature, problems with inflectional morphology can occur. For this reason, inflectional morphology is included in most assessments of grammatical aspects of language, while derivational is not.

Inflectional morphology in English is comparatively restricted compared with that of many other European languages. For this reason it has proved possible to include this aspect of morphology together with the full range of syntactic structures on the LARSP chart (see below).

If we turn our attention to syntax, we can identify three levels of sentence analysis: firstly the role of the sentence itself, for example whether it is a statement, a question, or a command. Secondly, we can examine the clause level: that is identify the clause elements within the sentence. Clause elements are the major building blocks of sentences, and comprise of categories such as Subject, Verb, Object, Complement and Adverbial. We will illustrate these further below in our discussion of LARSP.

Finally, we can analyse the lowest sentence level: the phrase level. This is the level where we classify what groups of words can be used to make up the clause elements. For example, in a sentence such as "Fred saw Freda", the Subject ("Fred"), the Verb ("saw") and the Object ("Freda") comprise of a single word each; however, in a sentence such as "the tall, thin, grey-haired man was watching the woman in the green coat", we see that the phrase level of English syntax allows other combinations of words to act as Subject ("the tall, thin, grey-haired man"), Verb ("was watching") and Object ("the woman in the green coat"). Again, we will look at this further in the section on LARSP.

5.1 Morpheme Analysis
There exist several language analysis techniques that rely solely on an analysis of morphemes, most of which are based on Brown's (1973) investigation of the mean length of utterance (MLU) in morphemes in children's speech. According to this approach, different stages of linguistic development in young children correlate closely to the MLU in morphemes found in a representative sample. Therefore, an MLU score will give a good idea of which linguistic stage the child is operating at (see Brown, 1973, for an account of the different linguistic stages).

Most of the techniques based on MLU devote a considerable amount of space to guidance on identifying different morphemes. These include Bloom and Lahey (1978), Miller (1981), and Stickler (1987). To give an example of the guidance given in such accounts, we include here some of Chapman's (1981) rules (based in turn on Brown, 1973).

> Stuttered repetitions are counted as a single morpheme, but deliberate repetitions (e.g. for emphasis) are counted separately.
> Fillers such as *mm* or *oh* are not counted, but *no*, *yeah*, and *hi* are.
> All compound words (two or more free morphemes), proper

names, and ritualized reduplications count as single words.

All irregular pasts of the verb (*got, did, went, saw*) count as one morpheme. There is no evidence that the child relates these to present forms.

All diminutives (*doggie, mommie*) count as one morpheme because children do not seem to use the suffix productively.

All auxiliaries count as separate morphemes.

All inflections count as separate morphemes.

Chapman also notes various features (such as amount of repetition or imitation) which might affect MLU.

An MLU score needs to be interpreted in terms of language development in order to be of use to the speech-language pathologist. However, Brown (1973) pointed out that MLU is only a general indicator of structural development, and is only reliable when it falls between 1.01 and 4.49. The table reproduced at the end of this section from Chapman (1981) shows the relation between Brown's (1973) language stages, MLU, and chronological age (this last computed by Miller and Chapman, 1979, in Chapman, 1981).

Chapman also notes that a distributional analysis of MLU can be undertaken (perhaps as a preliminary to the ASS procedure: see section 3 below). This provides for an analysis of which utterances from the sample showed an MLU of one morpheme, two morphemes, etc. In this way different syntactic structural types can be linked to different MLUs. Such an analysis can also be used to work out the number of utterances per speaker turn which can then be used as an input to pragmatic analyses.

Most who work with MLU measurements recognise that this approach can only be used as part of a wider investigation of linguistic structures. Indeed, profiles such as LARSP (see the following section) include details on specific inflectional morphemes along with an analysis of syntax. In effect, it combines in one process what with MLU measures takes two (i.e. the analysis of morphemes, and the relationship of this to structural stages). MLU is no longer such a popular measure as it once was, but it can still prove useful as a preliminary, screening procedure.

Brown's stages	MLU	predicted age
early Stage I	1.01	19.1
	1.10	19.8
	1.20	20.6
	1.30	21.4
	1.40	22.2
	1.50	23.0
late Stage I	1.60	23.8
	1.70	24.6
	1.80	25.3
	1.90	26.1
	2.00	26.9
Stage II	2.10	27.7
	2.20	28.5
	2.30	29.3
	2.40	30.1
	2.50	30.8
Stage III	2.60	31.6
	2.70	32.4
	2.80	33.2
	2.90	34.0
	3.00	34.8
early Stage IV	3.10	35.6
	3.20	36.3
	3.30	37.1
	3.40	37.9
	3.50	38.7
late Stage IV -	3.60	39.5
early Stage V	3.70	40.3
	3.80	41.1
	3.90	41.8
	4.00	42.6
late Stage V	4.10	43.4
	4.20	44.2
	4.30	45.0
	4.40	45.8
	4.50	46.6

Brown's stages	MLU	predicted age
post Stage V	4.60	47.3
	4.70	48.2
	4.80	48.9
	4.90	49.7
	5.00	50.5
	5.10	51.3
	5.20	52.1
	5.30	52.8
	5.40	53.6
	5.50	54.4
	5.60	55.2
	5.70	56.0
	5.80	56.8
	5.90	57.5
	6.00	58.3

5.2 LARSP

The Language Assessment Remediation Screening Procedure (LARSP) was the first of the collection of linguistic profiles for language disorders that have been produced in recent times, and which are the focus of this book. The first version was published in Crystal, Fletcher and Garman (1976), with the current version being included in Crystal (1982), and in the second edition of Crystal, Fletcher and Garman (1989). This profile has proved popular among speech pathologists for a variety of disorders appearing often in the clinical linguistics literature (see for example, Crystal, 1979), and versions for other languages have also been drawn up (see review in Ball, 1988a).

As with most of the profiles reviewed in this volume, the input for the LARSP procedure should normally be natural speech data (spontaneous and guided where possible) recorded by the speech pathologist. It is, of course, possible to use language data obtained via some standard elicitation procedure, though the authors of LARSP are at pains to point out (as we did in Chapter 1) that such data are often neither comprehensive nor representative.

The language sample must be transcribed from the tape-recording before analysis can proceed. Normally, it is sufficient to transcribe the sample into ordinary orthography, though clearly IPA transcription may be needed to record pecularities of pronunciation, or utterances that are not clear. Following this step, the sample must be analysed on several syntactic and morphological levels, before the constructions used can be entered onto the LARSP chart. Before we look at the chart in any detail (the LARSP Chart is reproduced at the end of this section), we will examine how this analysis takes place by using a typical piece of normal language.

If we had recorded the following utterance, we would need to make an analysis consisting of four steps: "the big dog had been eating the cat's dinner in the yard".

1. Sentence type: statement
2. Clause elements: {S(ubject) the big dog} {V(erb) had been eating} {O(bject) the cat's dinner} {A(dverbial) in the yard}
3. Phrase elements: S = determiner+adjective+noun; V = auxiliary+auxiliary+main verb; O = determiner+noun+noun; A = preposition+determiner+noun.
4. Inflectional affixes (word level): aspect marker on verb = eat+ing; past tense marker on auxiliary = had; past participle marker on auxiliary = been; genitive marker on noun = cat+'s.

This can be displayed as follows:

the big dog	had been eating	the cat's dinner	in the yard
S	V	O	A
D Adj N	aux aux vb	D N N	Pr D N
	ed en ing	's	

This sentence contains only one main verb, and this type is normally termed a "simple sentence"; "complex sentences" are those containing two or more main verbs (and therefore two or more clauses). When such sentences occur in a sample undergoing LARSP analysis, we need to extend the Clause Element level to account for them. Multi-clause sentences use two separate strategies to "add-on" the extra clauses: coordination and subordination. Coordination (the use of coordinators such as "and" or "but") involves the addition of a new, but independent, clause as in the example below:

Freda saw Fred but she didn't see Ferdy

    S   V   O   c   S   V   O

Subordination, on the other hand, involves converting one of the Clause elements of the "main clause" (S, O, C or A) into a clause through the use of subordinators such as "when", "because" "if" etc, as in the following example:

Freda saw Fred <u>when he was following Ferdy</u>

    S   V   O   A time

                    s   S   V   O

The LARSP chart allows the recording of both coordination and subordination as well as the other levels of analysis noted above.

Of course, in the sort of language samples we encounter in the clinic, we will often find constructions that are not what we would expect from normal adult speakers. Some of these differences will reflect simpler syntactic patterns characteristic of early stages in the acquisition of syntax, while others may be clearly deviant. In the LARSP procedure it is important to remember that error analysis is not the primary purpose of the analysis; clearly deviant syntax, therefore, is generally not analysed (unless a clear pattern emerges), while delayed syntactic patterns are entered onto the chart. One part of the chart is devoted to noting common examples of delayed syntax, but only within a developmental rather than an error scoring approach.

We can now turn attention to the layout of the LARSP chart itself. The top of the chart is for completing the normal information on the patient and sample. There is then a section on the interaction between therapist and patient. This in turn is divided into four sub-sections: A, where unanalysed and problematic utterances can be numbered; B, for an account of the types of response utterances used by the patient; C, for the types of spontaneous utterances used by the patient; and D, for an account of the therapist's reactions to the patient's utterances.

For sub-sections B and C there is the ability to mark when the patient uses ellipsis. Unfortunately, many previous language tests have not accounted for ellipsis (a very common, and quite natural phenomenon), demanding full responses only as correct. LARSP allows the therapist to note appropriate use of ellipsis in the patient's sample, and to note the amount of ellipsis used in each case.

Following this section is the main profile chart. This is designed with two main dimensions: grammatical categorization across the top of the chart, and developmental stages running down the left side. This combination works by placing specific grammatical constructions not only in the correct grammatical column, but also in the developmental role appropriate for its first expected use.

The very first line is devoted to the recording of minor sentences, such as responses (*yes, no*) and vocatives (*Mummy, Janey*). These emerge early on, but are of course retained; because of their special nature they cannot be analysed grammatically in the way major sentences are, and so are given this separate entry.

The remainder of the grammatical categories are for major sentences and the elements that make them up. LARSP divides major sentences firstly by sentence role: command, question and statement. For each of these types there are columns where the clause element information making them up is recorded. There is, however, a single phrase element column, into which the phrasal properties of the clause elements of all three sentence types are entered. The final column is for word level material, i.e. inflectional morphology. To the left of the clause level columns there is a column to record connectivity between clauses in terms of the coordinators and subordinators used.

This layout extends down the chart from developmental Stage I (0;9-1;6) to Stage V (3;0-3;6). We will return below to the make-up of the chart in the final two Stages. All the clause and phrase columns are divided into these five stages, but the word level column is not. This column extends from Stage II to V, and is left undivided for, according to the authors, although there is some agreement on the order the first few of these inflections emerge, there is no general agreement on age levels.

Stage I (0;9-1;6) is considered as the one-word stage, and

LARSP allows here only a basic analysis into, for example, verb-like units, or question-like units. It is only at Stage II (1;6-2;0) - the two-word stage - that true syntax begins to emerge. With commands, imperative verbs followed by another element (e.g. *go away!*) may occur; in questions we get the development of question-words together with another element (e.g. *where Mummy?/Mummy where?*). Likewise, two clause elements can now be found in statements, such as *me like* (SV), *Mummy dinner* (SO), or *eat biscuit/biscuit eat* (VO). It is worth noting here that, especially in the early stages, it is not unusual to get orders of elements that are different from the adult language. The authors of LARSP make it clear that abbreviations on the chart such VO stand just as much for OV, and are not intended to be prescriptive. If such changes in the orders of elements persist through later stages, they would naturally be considered as errors, and the chart allows for these to be noted. As is normally the case in profiles, an Other category is included for both Clause and Phrase columns at most stages.

The phrase level column at Stage II also lists two-word utterances, such as DN (*the house*), AdjN (*red car*), PrN (*in bus*) and Vpart (*turn off*). Clearly, some of these constructions will occur in more advanced language as part of clause elements in utterances longer than two words (e.g. *Daddy bought the house*); indeed, throughout the phrase element column this is of course going to happen. Nevertheless, LARSP requires that these phrasal combinations be entered at the relevant earlier stage. This is because it is the task of neither the phrase nor clause information to display how many words the child used per utterance, but to show the level of structures used. In fact, LARSP does allow us to see when the patient is moving from a simple one-word per clause element usage to something more sophisticated. Between Stages II and III, and III and IV there is a special transitional line divided off by dotted lines. Here there are abbreviations to show when an S, V, C, O or A element has been realised by more than one word. The categories here are additional to the main clausal categories which are still filled in. We can illustrate the use of this feature as follows: *Daddy bought the house* would be entered as SVO at the clause level, DN at the phrase level, and -ed at the word level (the single words *Daddy* and *bought* do not get entered at the phrase level, as they are too basic to need noting separately from their clause level entries). However, this utterance demonstrates a two-word O, so it will be entered on the Stage III-IV transitional liné as *XY*+O:NP, to be read as an utterance consisting of an Object plus two other clause elements has a Noun Phrase as the Object. If one utterance had S, V, and O (for example) realised by phrasal elements longer than a single word for all three, then three entries would be made on the appropriate transitional line.

Stage III (2;0-2;6) is the three-word stage. Here, in the command column, we would enter utterances such as *give that to me* (V*XY*), and *let* and *do* commands (*let me go, do be good*). In the question column we find longer q-word questions, and also the appearance of verb-first or yes-no questions (e.g. *is Daddy there?*). In the statement column we now find a large range of possible types including SVO (e.g. *Mummy sees dolly*), SVA (*Baby in playpen*), and VOA (*cooking dinner in kitchen*). At the phrase level we get both three-word phrasal construction such as DAdjN (*the red car*) and PrDN (*in the kitchen*), but also single-word phrasal elements that are important from a developmental viewpoint: the use of pronouns (personal and others), auxiliary verbs (modals and others), and the copula (e.g. the verb *to be* when not acting as an auxiliary). Examples of these include *I*, *me, you, their* (personal pronouns); *anyone, somewhere* (other pronouns); *can, may, must, shall, would* (modal auxiliaries); *be, have, do* (other auxiliaries). The development of these categories is important in the transition from very young speech styles, to more mature ones; it is clearly important, therefore, that they are specifically included on the LARSP chart.

Stage IV (2;6-3;0) is deemed to have clause elements of four-words or more. However, in the Command and Question columns we also get more advanced constructions that are not all of four elements. For example, we see commands including the subject (e.g *You open the door!*), as well as longer ordinary commands (V*XY*+ *give me the book now!*). For questions we see not only the development of longer q-word questions and yes-no questions, but also the stabilisation of verb before subject in q-word questions (e.g. *where is Daddy going?* instead of *where daddy is going?*), and the development of tag questions (*that's nice, isn't it?*).

Stage IV statements include various four element types, including SVOA (*Mummy saw Janey there*) and AA*XY* (*Daddy's going to town tomorrow*). At the phrase level there are various longer phrasal constructions, such as PrDAdjN (*in the red car*), but also phrasal negation (NegV *don't like*, Neg*X no cake*), phrasal coordination (*X*c*X cats and dogs*), and the use of two auxiliaries (*had been looking*).

Stage V (3;0-3;6) is a different type of stage, one called by the authors *recursion*. This involves the ability to construct complex sentences by connecting together clauses. This connectivity is shown in the Connectivity column, where the conjunctions used to join the clauses can be noted. Four main types are recognised: *and* (the most common connector in coordination), other coordinators (such as *but*, *or*), subordinators (such as *because, if, when, that, which, who* etc), and others (such as *well, so*). In the clause columns we are required only to mark that clausal connection has taken place, either of the coordination or subordination type. For the statement clause column (where more complexity is expected at this stage than with commands and questions), space is available to note whether the coordination/subordination comprises just two clauses or more than two; and for subordination, whether the subordinate clause is acting as A (the most common type) or S, C or O.

For the phrase level, we can mark postmodified clauses and phrases. Postmodified clause (sometimes termed *relative clauses*) diifer from subordinate clauses in that, instead of taking the place of an entire clause element, they act as postmodification in a noun phrase. We can illustrate this with the following two sentences:

I like <u>standing in the rain</u>
S V   O
             V   A

I like <u>the man {(who was) standing in the rain}</u>
S V   O
                               V   A = postmod cl

Postmodified phrases are similar, but lack the verb:

I like <u>the man {in the rain}</u>
S V   O
          D N Pr D N = postmod phr

The word level column ends at Stage V. As noted earlier, it is not divided between stages, but contains in probable chronological order (at least for the first affixes) the main inflectional affixes of English. These are the continuous aspect marker *-ing,* noun plural marker *pl*, past tense marker *-ed*, past participle marker *-en*, third singular present tense verb marker *3s*, genitive noun marker *gen*, abbreviated negative *n't*, abbreviated copula *'cop*, abbreviated auxiliary *'aux*, comparative and superlative adjective markers *-er*, *-est*, and adverb marker (strictly speaking a derivational affix) *-ly*. It should be noted that both regular and irregular forms are marked here, and even if the incorrect regular form is used for an adult irregular (or vice versa) it is marked here (and noted as incorrect elsewhere). For the three abbreviated types, it should be noted that this abbreviation should also be marked in the phrase column as an example of negative or copula or auxiliary.

Stage VI (3;6-4;6) contains information on system completion. It is divided into two main columns: additions to the system (shown as (+)), and retained errors (shown as (-)). Three main categories of addition are noted: noun phrase level (for example the use of the initiator, as in *all of the people were there*), verb phrase level (complex verb phrases of more than two auxiliaries: *we should have been watching*), and clause level, including passives (e.g. *we had been watched*).

The retained errors section is designed to show the sort of errors that should be being eradicated in the normal speech of a child at this age. It can, of course, be used for patients of whatever developmental level to record errors if this is what is required. However, it should be noted, that if a patient is operating at a level of Stage II to Stage IV, it is probably less profitable to record errors than abilities. Once, through therapy, the patient has reached the Stage VI level, then remaining errors can be concentrated on.

The errors are also divided into types. Errors in the use of clausal connectivity, clause elements, determiners, prepositions, pronouns and auxiliaries, and in inflectional morphology. Where necessary, specific error types are labelled: such as deletion or wrong word order. For the inflections, it is possible to mark, for both nouns, and verbs, whether an irregular ending has been used for a regular or vice versa.

The final stage, Stage VII (4;6+) allows a relatively small space to describe features of language development beyond the basic system. It has boxes for features of discourse (including empty subjects such as *it* in *it's raining*, and *there* in *there are a lot of people here*), syntactic comprehension, and style.

At the bottom of the chart should be filled in the total number of sentences in the sample, the mean number of sentences the patient used in each turn in the interaction with the therapist, and the mean length of sentences measured in words. This clearly gives us an insight into the patient's overall verbal abilities.

Once the chart has been completed, it is necessary to see how the profile aids in remediation. With language delayed patients, what we normally find in LARSP analyses is a chart where by and large the entries cease at some stage prior to that expected for the patient's age. This gives us a straightforward guide to intervention; in order to design a therapeutic program that follows the developmental norm, we must concentrate therapy on those clause and phrase level structures that follow on from where the patient's development has stopped. It is sometimes necessary to go back first, and clear up any structures from earlier stages that appear to have been by-passed, but apart from that, the aim must be to progress the patient down the chart until their linguistic development matches the norm for their age (in the case of any patient over about 5;0, that will be of course the effective end of the chart at Stage VI).

Name		Age	Sample date	Type

A	**Unanalysed**				**Problematic**		
	1 Unintelligible	2 Symbolic Noise	3 Deviant		1 Incomplete	2 Ambiguous	3 Stereotypes

B	**Responses**					Normal Response						Abnormal		
							Major							
				Repetitions	Elliptical			Reduced	Full	Minor	Structural	∅	Problems
	Stimulus Type	Totals			1	2	3+						
	Questions												
	Others												

C	**Spontaneous**

D	**Reactions**		General	Structural	∅		Other	Problems

Stage I (0;9–1;6)

Minor		Responses			Vocatives	Other	Problems
Major	Comm.	Quest.		Statement			
	'V'	'Q'	'V'	'N'	Other		Problems

Stage II (1;6–2;0)

Conn.		Clause				Phrase		Word
	VX	QX	SV	AX	DN	VV	
			SO	VO	Adj N	V part	-ing
			SC	VC	NN	Int X	pl
			Neg X	Other	PrN	Other	

Stage III (2;0–2;6)

	X + S:NP	X + V:VP	X + C:NP	X + O:NP	X + A:AP	
	VXY	QXY	SVC	VCA	D Adj N	Cop	-ed
	let XY		SVO	VOA	Adj Adj N		-en
		VS(X)	SVA	VO₀ρ,	Pr DN	Aux$_0^M$	3s
	do XY	Neg XY	Other	Pron₀'	Other		gen

Stage IV (2;6–3;0)

	XY + S:NP	XY + V:VP	XY + C:NP	XY + O:NP	XY + A:AP	
	+ S	QVS	SVOA	AAXY	NP Pr NP	Neg V	n't
		QXY +	SVCA	Other	Pr D Adj N	Neg X	'cop
	VXY +	VS(X+)	SVO₀ρ,		cX	XAux	'aux
		tag	SVOC		XcX	Other	

Stage V (3;0–3;6)

and	Coord.	Coord.	Coord.	1	1+	Postmod. 1 clause	1 +	-est
c	Other	Other	Subord. A	1	1 +			-er
s			S	C	O	Postmod. 1+ phrase		-ly
Other			Comparative					

	(+)				(−)	

Stage VI (3;6–4;6)

	NP	VP	Clause	Conn.	Clause		Phrase				Word	
					Element	NP			VP		N	V
	Initiator	Complex	Passive	and	∅	D	Pr	Pron'	Aux^M	Aux^0 Cop	irreg	
	Coord.		Complement.	c	⇌	D∅	Pr∅					
			how what	s	Concord	D ⇌	Pr ⇌		∅		reg	
	Other								Ambiguous			

Stage VII (4;6+)

Discourse			Syntactic Comprehension	
A Connectivity	it			
Comment Clause	there		Style	
Emphatic Order	Other			

Total No. Sentences	Mean No. Sentences Per Turn	Mean Sentence Length

© D. Crystal, P. Fletcher, M. Garman. 1981 revision, University of Reading

5.2 ASS/CSD

Assigning Structural Stage (ASS, Miller, 1981) together with its related procedure Analyzing Complex Sentence Development (CSD, Paul, 1981) is claimed to be a straightforward procedure to provide a detailed description of a child's structural development in syntax. Like LARSP, the procedure has a developmental metric, and requires an analysis of the syntax of the patient. However, it is unlike LARSP in that it does not consist of a single standard chart (or set of charts), with a single way of proceeding. As Miller points out, "there is no right way to carry out this procedure" (p31); he does, however, present guidelines which have proved useful to other clinicians.

The aim of the procedure is to assign various morphological and syntactic structures to stages of development to obtain an overall stage assignment for the patient, which can then be compared to the child's age and MLU. From this it can be determined whether the child's syntax is delayed or not.

The initial step recommended is the 14 morpheme analysis. This is not simply an analysis of inflectional morphemes, but also includes a sub-set of function words; the whole set being representative of Stages II to V+ of the Brown (1973) system. The following table lists these 14 morphemes.

stage	morpheme
II	*-ing*
	plural
	in
III	*on*
	possessive
V	regular past
	irregular past
	regular 3rd person singular
	articles *a, the*
	contractible copula *be*
V+	contractible auxiliary *be*
	uncontractible *be*
	irregular 3rd person singular

Following this part of the analysis, the Structural Development Charts can be tackled. These charts (which are too long to reproduce here, see Miller, 1981, p55-65 for ASS, and 67-71 for CSD) are in fact sets of examples of various structures together with the stage and MLU at which the structures are expected to emerge. The ASS charts are divided into six main categories: single-word utterances, noun phrase, verb phrase, negation, yes-no questions, and wh-questions; finally, it is recommended that a summary ASS worksheet is drawn up for each patient listing the structures to be concentrated on (see example at the end of this section, from Miller, 1981). In relation to this, Miller points out that it is not always necessary to analyse every possible construction, and that not every construction the child uses is listed on the charts which are restricted to those constructions for which the author had developmental data. This contrasts with the LARSP approach, which demands an analysis of all unproblematic utterances, and attempts a high degree of comprehensiveness in the structures listed.

The final stage in this process is the determination of overall stage assignment. Two different ways of working this out are suggested. Firstly, the analyst can assign a stage to each construction type (i.e. noun phrase, verb phrase, etc, according to the ASS charts). The stage assignment that occurs most often across the range of construction types is then chosen to summarize the stage of usual performance. A second method is to derive an overall score reflecting best ability, by averaging out the highest stage scores across the construction types. Clearly combining these two methods could give us a double score: that of usual performance, and that of newly acquired constructions. Indeed, this combination is useful in determining whether children are in fact still progressing in syntactic development, or whether this development is blocked. Miller concludes (p36) that "the examination of ASS data gives us more than just a stage assignment. It allows us to interpret the child's performance and to infer strengths and weaknesses that will be relevant in prescribing a syntactic therapy program".

ASS Summary Worksheet

Name:		MLU:	Age:		Date:
			Number of utterances:		
Stage	Noun phrase elaboration	Verb phrase elaboration		Negatives	Questions
I	NP → (M)+N alone only:	unmarked verb: absent aux: absent copula:		no/not + NP/VP	Wh: routines: *what, what do, where*
II	(M)+N in object position:	main verb marked: *-ing* without *be*: catenative alone: copula appears:		Neg→ *no, not* *can't, don't*	Wh: novel:
III	NP → demon/art+(M)+N demonstratives: *a, the* appear: quantifiers: possessives: adjectives:	pres.aux: *can, will, be*: overgen'l of *-ed*:		*won't*	Wh: aux appears without inversion *why, who, how* yes/no: rising intonation:
IV	NP → demon/art/(M)/poss+ adj+N:	main V and aux doubly marked for past in neg: past modals: catenative+NP: *be+-ing*:		Neg → pres *be*, *can, will, do, did, does*:	Wh: *do* appears: aux: inverted: *when*: yes/no: aux inverted: *do* appears:
V		V+: past *be*: *have +-en*:		Neg → past *be*, past modals:	

71

The CSD procedure is basically similar to that of ASS, but is concerned with complex sentences, i.e. those containing more than one verb (and so more than one clause). Two main clause types are identified: conjoined clauses and embedded clauses (corresponding more or less to the coordination/subordination dichotomy of LARSP). Surprisingly, perhaps, clauses introduced by *before* or *after* are counted as conjoined clauses, when to many linguists these would be simply examples of subordination based on adverbial elements.

As with ASS, these complex sentence types are listed together with information on normal stage development, and an overall stage assignment can be worked out using also information from the 14 morpheme analysis and the ASS data.

In many ways ASS/CSD and LARSP are similar. Both assign developmental values to particular syntactic stages, and both require an analysis of the patient's syntax, rather than the ability to respond to set elicitation procedures. However, LARSP perhaps has the advantage for several reasons: it has a straightforward one-page chart, it is comprehensive in its categories and its analysis, and it does not require the complicated methods of stage assignment.

5.3 Other Profiles
There have been developed numerous tests and assessment procedures for syntax, and we only have the space to mention briefly just a few of these that seem to us to follow most closely the guidelines for profiles laid down in Chapter 1.

Lee (1974) developed the *Developmental Sentence Types* and *Developmental Sentence Scoring* procedures for spontaneous discourse, using as input the first 100 (for *DST*) and the first 50 (for *DSS*) utterances of a sample. With *DST*, various types of basic presentence are recognized, and constructions such as noun phrase, prepositional phrases and various clause types can be noted. The procedure is unlike LARSP, but similar to ASS/CSD, in that clinicians are urged to adapt the it to suit their purposes. For *DSS*, scores are assigned for particular constructions, and then compared with normative scores.

Tyack and Gottsleben's (1974) *Language Sampling, Analysis, and Training (LSAT)* also uses the first 100 sentences of a sample of spontaneous speech. The patient's level is worked out by computing the mean number of words as a ratio of the mean number of morphemes per sentence. This level corresponds to a linguistic stage where particular structures are to be expected. The various structures at these stages can be checked against the patient's performance, and so therapy goals can be established.

Stickler's (1987) *Guide to Analysis of Language Transcripts* has a section on syntactic analysis (it also covers morphology, and pragmatics). This approach is in fact simply a slightly more directed version of ASS/CSD, and needs no further comment here.

Lund and Duchan (1987) also provide a guide to the analysis of syntax. Like Crystal, Fletcher and Garman (1976, 1989), they provide an account of syntax and a description of syntactic development, and aim to combine the two to provide their syntactic analysis. They include a series of worksheets where numbered utterances can be transcribed, but the system lacks the compactness of the LARSP chart, and the comprehensiveness of description.

In recent times, various computerized syntactic analyses have appeared. LARSP, for example, exists in computerized form (see Long, 1987, Long and Fey, 1990a,b, and Long and Long, 1990). A derivative of the LARSP procedure for computers is CLEAR (*Computerised Language Error Analysis Report*, Baker-van den Goorbergh and Baker, 1991), described also in Baker-van den Goorbergh (1990). This system not only aids in the analysis of the data, but also provides a range of graphic displays and printouts to summarize clearly the analyst's results.

However, one of the first computerized syntactic analysis systems was SALT (*Systematic Analysis of Language Transcripts*) devised by Miller and Chapman (1985), where the clinician codes the syntactic structures encountered in a sample of spontaneous speech, and summaries of the structures are produced by the program. Long and colleagues have produced a variety of computer packages combining a version of SALT with other procedures such as LARSP, DSS for syntax, and other procedures for semantics, pragmatics and phonology (see especially Long and Fey, 1990a,b). These programs now run on a variety of hardware and clearly will be of use to clinicians proficient in personal computing.

Finally, we can also mention Pye's (1987) *PAL* (see also Pye and Ingram, 1988). The *Pye Analysis of Language* contains programs for analysing the productivity of a child's rules in different areas of language. Available are measures of word frequencies, phonetic frequencies and substitutions, MLU, and a lexical and syntactic concordance.

Chapter 6

SEMANTICS

Introduction

Semantics is the linguistic term for the study of meaning. However, this area of linguistic investigation has proved much less tractable than syntax or phonology, for example. One, over-arching, theory of meaning has not been achieved, and it is debateable as to whether such a theory could ever be built.

Nevertheless, meaning-related disorders are important in many types of language pathology, and it is essential, therefore, that semantics is not excluded from our consideration just because it is difficult to analyse and assess.

Of course, all parts of the linguistic code contribute to the meaning that the hearer extracts from an utterance; however, it can be argued that semantics can profitably be examined primarily from two perspectives. The first of these is concerned with individual word meaning (lexical semantics), while the second is concerned with words in context, i.e. the meaning roles found in sentences (grammatical semantics).

In the context of disordered language, Crystal (1982) suggests that these two approaches can be viewed in slightly different ways. With lexical semantics, it is not only important to note whether particular words are used "correctly" or "incorrectly", but it is also necessary to produce a picture of the range of lexical items ($\simeq$ words, see below) that a client uses. This will be of use for both language delayed/disordered children, and for certain types of adult patient who may suffer from lexical erosion.

On the other hand, when we come to examine grammatical semantics, we need to make a record of the types and complexities of semantic sentence roles that the patient can use, and how correct these are, in much the same way as is done in syntactic analyses.

As noted above, semantics is an area which many linguistic

researchers have avoided: and the same is true of clinical linguists. In fact there are only two major semantic profiles, one devoted to lexical semantics (PRISM-L) and the other to grammatical semantics (PRISM-G), both first described in Crystal (1982). In order to understand better the approaches to profiling these areas, we will examine the two profiles in the following sections.

6.1 PRISM-L

One of the areas of study within lexical semantics is the examination of semantic fields. A semantic field is an area of meaning which will be expressed in the language concerned by a range of lexical items. We can give an example to show what we mean here: the semantic field of "animals" in English contains numerous lexical items, including "cow", "pig" "sheep", "horse" "lion" "dog", "cat" etc. Of course, we might instead wish to take a smaller semantic field of "sheep", where we would find lexical items such as "ram", "ewe", "lamb", "wether", etc. The concept itself, then, is relatively fluid: the size of a semantic field (i.e. the range of meanings and possible lexical items covering them) is dependant on the amount of detail the researcher wishes to encompass.

The importance of such an approach to disordered language can be seen, for example, in the occurrence of semantic/lexical overgeneralization that is found in child language. Here, we often find one lexical item taking on the function of several (or, indeed, all) others in that semantic field. So, we may find "doggy" being used not only for "dog" but for all quadruped animals as well, thus covering "cat", "cow", "horse" and so on. Conversely, at early stages of development we can find undergeneralization, whereby the term is restricted to one individual only, and not used to cover a range as in adult usage. An example here might be when "doggy" is applied *only* to the family pet dog and not to other dogs.

While both over- and undergeneralization may be found clinically in language delayed children, patients suffering from a variety of acquired adult neurological disorders may also exhibit disturbances to their lexicons. These disturbances might also involve selective loss or disorder in different semantic fields, ranging from total deletion of some fields to minimal problems with others.

For several reasons, therefore, it can be important to investigate the lexical semantics (i.e. semantic fields) of a particular patient. The potential difficulty here lies with selective commentary. That is to say that if the clinician relies solely on noting examples as they happen to occur, the overall pattern of use will not emerge. However, the task of preparing a comprehensive description is a daunting one.

It is here that PRISM-L makes its contribution as a profile of vocabulary (see also Crystal, 1982). Like most of the other profiles we have looked at in this book, PRISM-L (PRofile In SeMantics - Lexical) relies for input on a recording of the spontaneous speech (where possible) of the patient. For semantic work this only needs transcribing into normal orthography.

The analysis is one of lexemes (= lexical items) used by the patient. We can normally divide such items into two broad classes for the purposes of an analysis such as this. The first of these encompasses words that tend to occur with regularity in a sample. These will usually be what are often termed "functives" ("function words") such as articles, conjunctions, prepositions and pronouns, together with auxiliary verbs. For PRISM-L these are classed together as "minor lexemes" and if required can be entered onto the relevant page of the profile chart. Also included in this overall category is the social use of language, for example greetings, exclamations, responses, and proper names (see page 2 of the chart at the end of this section).

Remaining words should be categorized as major lexemes and entered onto the major lexemes part of the chart (pages 4-15 of the chart). This is divided into 63 main fields, most with several sub-fields noted. The fields themselves are not arranged arbitrarily, but follow a pattern. Initially this is broadly developmental with early sections reflecting early vocabulary acquisition. While later sections reflect more advanced vocabulary, no claim is made to any precise linear progression there.

The first two pages of the chart cover semantic fields in the area of human form and function, and the next two activity and the senses. These are followed by a page on leisure and one on transport; then fauna; flora and the elements; the domestic setting; dimensions; and a double page on institutions and the world (Crystal, 1982, p150). Naturally, although wide-ranging, one cannot expect to cover all areas of vocabulary in a schema such as this, therefore the final section sees the essential "other" category.

Before going on to see how PRISM-L's material is summarized, we need to clarify the procedure whereby entries are calculated. So far we have used the terms "word" and "lexeme"/ "lexical item" without definition. PRISM-L deals in *'lexemes'* only - that is to say it is a type analysis rather than a token analysis. Let us illustrate this with the following example. The "lexeme" GO (lexemes are often represented in capitals) is a type; it may be realised by a number of different "words", such as "go", "goes", "going", "went", "gone". For entry on the PRISM-L chart any tokens of these five words would all be grouped together as tokens of one lexeme: GO. They would be entered on page 6 of the chart (third page of the major lexemes section), in the Field *Moving*, sub-field *come/go*. If one example each of "go", "goes", "going", "went", "gone" occurred in the data we would enter this as: *go* 5. This, however, would not be differentiated from five examples of, say, "going". That is because this is a semantic profile, not a morphological/syntactic one (LARSP would be where such differences could be made explicit), and we are investigating how well people can use semantic concepts.

Apart from an analysis into semantic fields, the lexical aspects of semantics can also cover relationships between lexical items, over- and undergeneralisations (as discussed earlier) and mistakes in the use of lexemes. All these features are covered on the last page of the profile chart. The first section covers "paradigmatic relations" such as synonyms and antonyms; the second "syntagmatic relations" such as idiomatic phrases; and the third developmental errors such as overextension and underextension, and mismatch: when the patient's word is clearly unconnected with the expected target (e.g. when "doggy" is used for expected target "house"). For the first two sections the chart allows the clinician to fill in both correct and incorrect usages.

PRISM-L, of course, presents a large amount of information which needs to be summarized. The first page of the profile chart aims to do this. It allows for up to 7 different samples, nicely providing for longitudinal studies/records, and information on the length and type of language data collected. Then for both minor and major lexemes it allows the clinician to note the number of types (lexemes) and tokens (words) and the ratio between them (giving an idea of the breadth of a patient's semantic range and the amount of lexeme repetition present). Further, for major lexemes, the number of semantic fields and sub-fields used can be noted.

As stated above, except in a minor way this profile is unlike LARSP in that it is not developmentally assessed. Nevertheless, the considerable time needed to input data to this profile is paid back for lexically disordered patients by the clear picture given of vocabulary breadth and semantic range.

6.2 PRISM-G

We commented earlier that other approaches to semantics, apart from the lexical, can be taken. An important alternative approach for the clinical linguist involves the investigation of the semantic roles used by a speaker in sentence production, and is termed in Crystal (1982) "grammatical semantics". To give an illustration of this field of study, and how it differs from an analysis into syntactic roles, we can consider the following sentences:

1. Fred was attacking Freda and Ferdy
2. Freda and Ferdy were attacked by Fred

In sentence 1 [Fred] is the syntactic subject (the verb agrees with the subject, as they are both singular), while in sentence 2 [Freda and Ferdy] is the subject (the verb agrees with the subject, as they are both plural). However, if we examine the semantic roles of these sentences and try to isolate the entity that "does" the action (the *actor*, also termed *agent*), and the entity affected by the action (the *goal*, also termed the *affected*), we find that in both sentence 1 and 2, [Fred] is the actor, and that in both sentence 1 and 2 [Freda and Ferdy] is the goal.

PRISM-L
Summary

Name		Age		Date of birth			
Sample no.							
Date							
Duration							
Type							
Unanalysed							
Minor (p.2) Types							
Tokens							
TTR							
Minor major (Tokens)							
Major (pp.4-5) Types							
Tokens							
TTR							
Fields used							
Sub-fields used							
Repetitions							
Comments							

PRISM-L
Minor Lexemes (Summary)

	Unanalysed	Unintelligible	Ambiguous	Symbolic Noise	Other
Social		Spontaneous		Response	
		Stereotype		Comment	
		Proper N		Other	
Relational		Pronominal 1 2 3		Dem Art Other	
		Prepositional Loc		Temp	Other Problems
		Verbal be 1 2 3		Other	Neg
		Interrogative		Tags	
		Connective			
		Empty		Other	
Avoidance					

PRISM–L
Major Lexemes (Summary)

Page					Totals	Ty			
						To			

Page								
4	Man	Body			Health			
5	Clothing							
6	Moving	Making/Doing	Food					
6	Having	Thinking		Happening	Living			
7	Sound	Sight		Feeling				
7		Smell	Taste	Touch				
7	Language		Imagination					
8	Recreation	Occasions	Shows	Music	Art			
9	Road	Rail	Air	Water	Fuel			
10	Animals	Birds	Fish	Insects				
11	Flowers	Trees	Light					
12	Colour	Fire	Water					
12	Building	Furniture	Tools	Containers				
13	Quantity	Measurement	Size	Shape				
13	Time	Location	State					
14	Government	Law	Education	Religion	Business	Manufacture		
15	Space	World	Minerals	Weapons	Money			
15	Other							

PRISM–L
Lexeme Inventory (Major Items)

Man				
	Family		Type	
	Jobs		General	
	Group		Contacts	
	Location		Other	
	Character +	–	Neutral	

Body				
	Main Parts		Limbs	
	Face		Outside	
	Health		Inside	
	Character +	–	Neutral	
	Other			

Health			
	Disease		
	People		Protection
	Other		Implements

81

PRISM-L

Moving	Come/Go	Static		Sleep	Animate
	Things	Other			
Making/Doing	General	Specific		Type	
Happening					Other
Living					Other
Having	Process +	Process −			
Thinking	Process	General		Type	Other
Feeling	+	−		Neutral	Other

PRISM-L

Clothing	General	Material		Outer	Footwear
	Man	Woman	Neutral	Child	
	Accessories	Parts		Caring	Other
Food (Grown)	Fruit	Part	Location		
	Vegetables	Grain	Part		
	Character	Other			
(Processed)	Type	Dairy	Seafood		
	Drinks	Flavouring			
Food (Grown and processed)	Action	Location			
	Meals	Utensils			
	People	Other			

PRISM-L

Sound	General	Specific	Quality		Other
Sight	Act		Implements		Other
Smell	Act		Character		Other
Taste	Act		Character		Other
Touch	Act		Character		Other
Language	Speak/Listen		Read/Write		Other
	Act	People	Pet	Product	Character	Other
Imagination	Type		People	Character	Other

PRISM-L

Recreation	Action		Location	
	Games		Sports	
	People		Equipment	
	Things		Other	
Occasions	General	X'mas	Location	Other
Shows	Type		Location	
Music	Instruments		Type	
	Action		People	
	Parts	Other		
Art	Implements		People	Type	Other
	Quality			

83

PRISM-L

Animals	General	Pet
	Farm	Wild(Small)
	Water	Wild (Large)
	Reptile	Extinct/Imaginary
	Noise	Location
	Action (Us → Them)	(Them → Us)
	Type	Parts	Other
Birds	Type	Parts
	Water	Farm
	Action	Noise	Other
Fish	Type	Parts
	Action	Control	Other
Insects	Type	Parts
	Action	Location	Other

PRISM-L

Land (Road)	Vehicle	Parts
	Action	Location
	People	Other
(Rail)	Vehicle	Parts
	Action	Location
	People	Other
Air	Vehicle	Parts
	Action	Location
	People	Other
Water	Vehicle	Parts
	Action	Location
	People	Other
Fuel		Other

PRISM-L

			Parts	
Flowers (etc.)	Type			
	Action		Other	
Trees	Type		Parts	
	Action		Other	
Light	Type		Control	Other
	Action		Implement	Other
Colour	Type		General	Other
Fire	Type		Fuel	
	Control		Other	
Water	Type		Action	
	Control		Other	

PRISM-L

		Parts	
Building	Type		
	Outside	Materials	
	Action	People	
	Rooms	Other	
Furniture	General	Bedroom	Living Room
	Kitchen/Dining	Other	
Tools	General	Farm/Garden	
	People	Other	
Containers	Type	Parts	
	Action	Other	

85

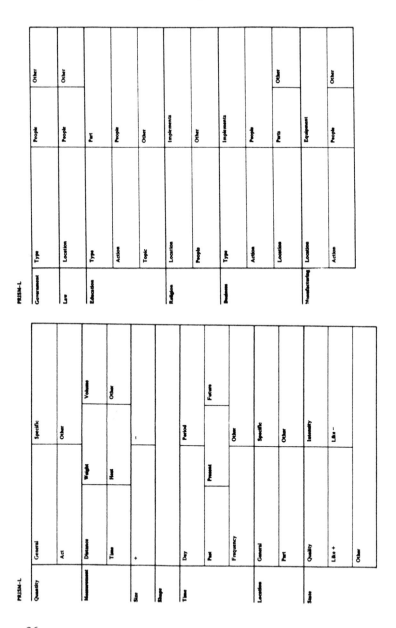

PRISM-L

	Entities/Events			Exploration	Other
Space					
World	Land	Surface		Water	Other
		Location	Climate	Depth	
Minerals	Type	Act			Other
Weapons	Type		People		Other
Money	Units		Location		Other
Memory	Action	Type			Other
Other					

PRISM-L
Further Analysis

	Synonymy	Error
Paradigmatic Relations	Opposition	
	Hyponymy	
	Incompatibility	
	Other	
Syntagmatic Relations		
	Other	
Developmental Error	Overextension	
	Underextension	
	Mismatch	

It is the aim of PRISM-G to profile a patient's use of such semantic roles, and like LARSP the profile chart is divided into stages that are basically developmental, though no set age ranges are identified here as our knowledge of this area is currently insufficient to allow precise figures. Also like LARSP is the facility to record at the head of the chart details of the patient and sample, and types of unanalysed utterances.

Crystal (1982) proposes a set of semantic roles to be used in the PRISM-G assessment, but readers should bear in mind that other approaches to semantics may well use more categories, and different names for them. In order to facilitate the move between the LARSP parsing procedure and that for PRISM-G, it can be noted that one set of semantic role terms is reserved for the main clausal elements of a LARSP type analysis (the semantic *elements*), while another set is used to classify the phrasal categories of LARSP (the semantic *specifiers*). Indeed, the concept of *minor* versus *major* elements is also retained, though the remaining discussion here deals only with the latter.

We will note most of the important semantic elements here (see also Crystal, 1982, p173): *actor* is an animate being causing a particular action or change (see our examples in sentences 1 and 2 above); *experiencer* is again an animate being that experiences the action or change of state (for example **Fred** *is tired*; **Freda** *saw Fred*); *goal*, on the other hand, is the object or being that suffers the result of an action or change of state (like [Freda and Ferdy] in sentences 1 and 2 above). Activity or state is divided into two categories: *dynamic*, which encompasses observable activity or change of state such as *attack, move, walk*; *static* on the other hand covers non-observable activity or change of state: *see, understand, think*. The final elements have to do with the placing of the meaning in space and time: *locative* (e.g. *Fred saw Freda* **in the park**); and *temporal* (e.g. *Ferdy met Freda* **at three o'clock**).

At the early stages of development, short sentences only may be found, and in such circumstances the full range of semantic elements may be inappropriate. Therefore, the elements *activity* (covering both *dynamic* and *static*), and *entity animate/entity inanimate* (covering *actor, experiencer, goal, location*) are used. Interrogatives when used as one-word utterances are noted under *interrog* during the early stages. Finally, the term *deictic* is used throughout the chart to note particular words with a function of "pointing" to semantic notions such as time and place or to particular individuals. They can be cross-classified against the semantic elements (e.g. *actor* for *he, temporal* for *now, locative* for *there*), but in the early stages are divided into *animate, inanimate* and *scope* (this latter covering the time and place meanings).

The semantic specifiers used in PRISM-G are as follows (see Crystal, 1982, p173): *scope*, items like prepositions specifying location, time, manner, purpose etc (*Freda saw Ferdy in the park*); *attribute* covers adjectives and the adjectival use of nouns (*Fred is a stupid idiot*); *definiteness* covers the use of determiners such as the articles and the demonstratives (*in the park*); *possessive* covers possessive adjectives and genitive nouns (*my car; Ferdy's house*); finally *quantity* is used to classify numerals and other expressions of amount (*two cars; some cars*). For both specifiers and elements there are of course "other" categories.

To fill in the form, one follows very much the same procedure as with LARSP, i.e. the recording of naturalistic speech data, its transcription (of course one set of data and its transcription could well serve as input to several profiles if needed), its analysis into elements and specifiers, and then entry onto the chart. The chart differs from LARSP in one respect, however, in that for most of the stages one can cross-classify the elements with the specifiers. As can be seen on the chart at the end of this chapter, as one part of each stage the elements are set in columns and the specifiers in rows, so that any element that also has a specifier can be noted in this part of the stage. A separate part is reserved for noting the element structure of an utterance itself. Finally, a separate box is also reserved for the deictic terms which can also be marked against the columns for elements. A special box at each stage allows the noting of interrogatives.

The first four stages of PRISM-G can be summarized through making use of the summary boxes provided at each stage. These record number of clauses, number of semantic elements, number of specifiers, and the number of deictic terms. Totals for all stages can be worked out, and from these we can discover the number of semantic elements the patient uses per clause, the number of specifiers per element, and the number of deictic terms per element. This information clearly gives us a picture of the range of semantic roles the speaker is able to manipulate in natural speech.

The final stage of the chart (V), concerns the semantics of multi-clause sentences (in the same way that stage V of LARSP concerns the syntax of multi-clause sentences) (see Crystal, 1982, p186f). The main part of this stage is a matrix showing the combination of various clauses (ranging from clauses with one semantic element each, to those with four or more in one and three or more in the other). These are plotted against eight different semantic linkages (plus of course an "other" category). These are *addition* (e.g. the use of *and*); *reformulation* (*or*); *contrast* (*but*); *temporal* (e.g. *when, after, before, while*); *cause* (e.g. *because, since*); *location* (e.g. *where*); *condition* (e.g. *if, although, whether*); and *purpose* (e.g. *to, so (that)*).

Stage V also allows the recording of *order of mention*, that is to say the correlation between the order of clauses and the order of events referred to. As an example, we can consider the following:

3. Fred saw Freda before he met Ferdy
4. Fred met Ferdy after he saw Freda

In sentence 3 the order of the clauses reflects the order of the actions, whereas in 4 the orders are reversed. It can be important to note orderings such as these, as problems are often encountered with language disordered patients with the reverse order of sentences such as in 4.

Another aspect of semantics recorded in this final section concerns what, broadly, might be termed ellipsis in the study of syntax. That is to say, especially in discourse, we often omit material that is known to the conversational partners, and might indeed have formed part of the previous utterance: e.g. *where are you going? - [I'm going] to town.* On PRISM-G such omissions are counted as *presupposed T elements*, i.e. elements that are missing because they were supplied by the therapist.

The final two sections of the PRISM-G chart are to note idiomatic expressions that are not susceptible to semantic element analysis, and an error box to note down utterances which, while they can be analysed, seem to be clear semantic errors (not simply syntactic or morphological, however). Crystal (1982, p194) gives the following as an example of idiomatic usage: *I take pleasure in reading*, and the following as an example of a semantic error: *see a man and a garage go.*

Semantics is clearly a difficult area both to analyse and to assess. However, a wide range of patients present with semantic disorders, and it clearly possible, using the two profiles we have looked at in this chapter, to undertake adequate assessments of both lexical and grammatical aspects of meaning. While both these procedures are time consuming, it is worth noting that computerizeed profiling does exist for PRISM-L (see Long, 1987), which will radically shorten the procedure. Long and Fey (1990) also report on another computerized semantic analysis: APRON, for relational semantic analysis. See also Lund and Duchan (1987) for descriptions of other semantic analyses.

PRISM-G	Name	Age	Sample	Total

Unanalysed Unintelligible	Incomplete	Symbolic Noise	Ambiguous	Stereotypes	

I

Minor

Social	Proper Name	Other	+ Specifications

Major

Elements	Activity		Entity		Deictic				Attr	Inter-rog	Other
	Dyn	Stat	Anim	Inanim	Anim	Inanim	Sco	Other			
Cop											
+ Specification											
Scope											
Attribute											
Definiteness											
Possessive											
Quantity											
Other											

C/E

D

S

II

Elements	Act + Dyn	Exp + Stat	Poss + Stat	+ Interrog

	Dyn	Stat	Goal	Temp	Loc	Other
Dyn						
Stat						

	Ent	Attr	Temp	Loc	Other
Ent					

Other + Other	

+ Specification	Dyn	Stat	Act	Exp	Goal	Temp	Loc	Ent	Poss	Attr	Other
Scope											
Attribute											
Definiteness											
Possessive											
Quantity											
Other											

Deictic										

C

E

S

D

92

III

Elements	+ Goal	+ Temp	+ Loc	+ Other
Act + Dyn				
Exp + Stat				
Poss + Stat				
Dyn + Goal				
Stat + Goal				
Other				

+ Interrog

C

E

+ Specification	Dyn	Stat	Act	Exp	Poss	Goal	Temp	Loc	Other
Scope									
Attribute									
Definiteness									
Possessive									
Quantity									
Other									

S

D

Deictic								

IV

Elements	+ Temp	+ Loc	+ Other
Act + Dyn + Goal			
Exp + Stat + Goal			
Poss + Stat + Goal			
Other			

+ Interrog

C

E

+ Specification	Dyn	Stat	Act	Exp	Poss	Goal	Temp	Loc	Other
Scope									
Attribute									
Definiteness									
Possessive									
Quantity									
Other									

S

D

Deictic								

5+ Elements	

C   E

D   S

Deictic		+ Specification

Totals	Means
Major clauses (C)	Elements per clause (E/C)
Major elements (E)	Specifications per element (S/E)
Specifications (S)	Deictics per element (D/E)
Deictics (D)	

V

Unanalysed

Clause (A-B) Sequence

		Addition		Reform.		Contrast		Temporal		Cause		Location		Condition		Purpose		Other	
		Conn	∮	Conn	∮	Conn	∮	Conn	∮	Conn	∮	Conn	∮	Conn	∮	Conn	∮	Conn	∮
1 + 1	✓																		
	✗																		
1 + 2	✓																		
	✗																		
1 + 3⁺	✓																		
	✗																		
2 + 1	✓																		
	✗																		
2 + 2	✓																		
	✗																		
2 + 3⁺	✓																		
	✗																		
3 + 1	✓																		
	✗																		
3 + 2	✓																		
	✗																		
3 + 3⁺	✓																		
	✗																		
4⁺ + 1	✓																		
	✗																		
4⁺ + 2	✓																		
	✗																		
4⁺ + 3⁺	✓																		
	✗																		

Order-of-mention

	$C_1 \rightarrow C_2$	$C_1 \rightarrow C_2 \rightarrow C_3$	Other →	$C_2 \leftarrow C_1$	Other ←
✓					
✗					

Presupposed T elements

	1					2	3⁺	Clause
	Act/Exp	Dyn/Stat	Goal	Scope	Other			
✓								
✗								

Idiomatic

Error

Chapter 7

PRAGMATICS

Introduction

Pragmatics is a relatively new area of interest for linguists and for clinical linguists, nevertheless, if we look at the literature in this area it would seem that "clinical pragmatics" has suffered an explosive development in recent times. However, before we look at specific applications of pragmatics to assessing disordered language, we need to spend some time exploring what the term covers. Unfortunately, not all linguists agree as to the areas of study subsumed under the term pragmatics, with some preferring a "broad" interpretation, and others a "narrow" (see Leech, 1983, Levinson, 1983). For our purposes, however, we assume that the term covers all aspects of the communicative event which are not covered by the other levels of linguistics. This might include, therefore, features such as the rules of discourse or conversation, non-verbal behaviour, cohesion, fluency, and appropriate usage of sociolinguistic variation (see also Chapter 8). These features will become clearer when we examine the specific profiles of the following sections.

Disordered pragmatic behaviour is noted in a wide range of patients presenting in the speech-language pathology clinic, including children with speech-language delay, and adults with various types of acquired neurological disorders. Interestingly, it is the former that have prompted the majority of the large number of pragmatic assessments produced in recent times, while the latter have only very recently begun to provoke interest. Out of the large number of assessment procedures available, we have chosen to look in detail at two: one designed for children and adults, and one mainly for adult aphasics. While basically similar in their approach, they also display interesting differences that will be commented on. In our final section we list a range of other profiles and assessments.

7.1 Pragmatic Protocol

The Pragmatic Protocol was designed by Prutting and Kirchner (1983), and is shown here in its revised form of 1987. The Pragmatic Protocol chart is reproduced at the end of this section. Unlike some of the other profiles that we have examined, these pragmatic assessments operate more on the level of checklists of certain behaviours that may occur during a recording session, rather than profiles of sets of necessary building blocks to an adequate phonology or syntax. Further, whereas a profile such as LARSP has a developmental metric, the assessment of pragmatics is normally seen in terms of noting which behaviours are used "appropriately" and which "inappropriately". This clearly is a less exact way of measuring, as it opens a debate on how to measure appropriateness, and whether we are looking at this feature in terms of what a normal speaker would do, or what might be appropriate for a disordered speaker. This debate is opened in Ball, Davis, Duckworth and Middlehurst (in press), and we return briefly to the problem below.

The Pragmatic Protocol consists of thirty pragmatic parameters, divided into 7 groups, which in turn are assigned to three "aspects": verbal, paralinguistic, and non-verbal. The first of these is further divided into A. Speech Acts, B. Topic, C. Turn Taking, D. Lexical Selection and E. Stylistic Variation. Among the pragmatic parameters included here are variety of speech acts (A), topic selection. topic maintenance and topic change (B), initiation, response, repair, pause time, overlap, feedback, and adjacency (C), cohesion (D), and the varying of communicative style (E).

Paralinguistic Aspects contains only one section: F. Intelligibility and Prosodics. This in turn has five parameters: intelligibility, vocal intensity, vocal quality, prosody, and fluency. Finally, there is the Nonverbal Aspects, which also has only one division: G. Kenesics and Proxemics. This contains seven parameters: physical proximity, physical contacts, body posture, foot/leg and hand/arm movements, gestures, facial expressions, and eye gaze. While most of these parameters are fairly self-explanatory, readers are referred to Prutting and Kirchner (1983, 1987) for examples for those with which they are unfamiliar.

The chart contains these thirty parameters (following the space for the normal details of the patient and sample) set in a column at the left-hand side, with four columns ranging to the right for marking the profile. The two most important of these columns are the "Appropriate" and "Inappropriate" assessments; the others being "No opportunity to observe" and "Examples and comments". The authors provide specific guidance on assigning behaviours to either of the two main marking categories. This guidance is as follows:

> Appropriate. Parameters are marked appropriate if they are judged to facilitate the communicative interaction or are neutral.
>
> Inappropriate. Parameters are marked inappropriate if they are judged to detract from the communicative exchange and penalize the individual. (Prutting and Kirchner, 1987, p108).

The study reported in Prutting and Kirchner (1987) also reports on inter-scorer reliability (ranging between 91% and 100% for various groups of subjects); and on typical profiles for different language disorders.

7.2 PCA

This profile was devised by Penn (1988), based on earlier work (Penn, 1983). It was specifically designed for work with aphasics, and follows closely the analysis of pragmatics proposed in Levinson (1983). The profile chart is shown at the end of the section. The fifty or so parameters are grouped in six main sections: response to interlocutor, control of semantic content, cohesion, fluency, sociolinguistic sensitivity, and non-verbal communication.

Under response to interlocutor there are five main parameters: request, reply, clarification request, acknowledgement, teaching probe; under control of semantic content there are topic initiation, topic adherence, topic shift, lexical choice, idea completion and idea sequencing. The cohesion category contains seven main parameters: ellipsis, tense use, reference, lexical substitution forms, relative clauses, prenominal adjectives, and conjunctions; while the fluency section contains seven special categories: interjections, repetitions, revisions, incomplete phrases, false starts, pauses, and word-finding difficulties. Under sociolinguistic sensitivity we find polite forms, reference to interlocutor, placeholders and fillers, acknowledgements, self correction, comment clauses, sarcasm and humour, control of direct speech, and indirect speech acts. Finally, non-verbal communication contains two main sub-sections: vocal aspects (intensity, pitch, rate, intonation, and quality), and non-verbal aspects (facial expression, head movement, body posture, breathing, social distance, and gesture). Again, while most of these labels are self-explanatory, readers unsure of any terms are directed to Penn (1988).

It is interesting to note that while the two profiles have many parameters in common, there do not always organise these in the same way, and that there are differences in emphasis. The Pragmatic Profile, for example, puts a great stress on turn taking, while the PCA has more specifically linguistic categories in its sections on cohesion and fluency. These differences may reflect to some extent the fact that the PCA is specifically for adult patients, while the Protocol is aimed at both children and adults; but it also reflects the fact that in pragmatics (unlike syntax and phonology) there is not really any agreement on what constitute the basic units of the field of study.

Unlike the Protocol, the PCA requires a marking system using a five point scale: inappropriate, mostly inappropriate, some appropriate, mostly appropriate, appropriate, with a 'could not evaluate' category as well. Degree of appropriateness is measured against how far the behaviour interferes with conversational flow. This system clearly adds sensitivity to the analysis, but likewise could add to the difficulty in inter-scorer reliability. Statistical analysis reported in Penn (1988) suggests inter-scorer reliability in her investigation was good. She also reports on the diagnostic ability of the PCA, and is less strong in her claims than Prutting and Kirchner, noting that a wide range of pragmatic abilities may be affected in different ways by different patients even of the same overall aphasic type.

Pragmatic Protocol

NAME: _____   DATE: _____
COMMUNICATIVE   COMMUNICATIVE PARTNER'S
SETTING OBSERVED _____   RELATIONSHIP _____

Communicative act	Appropriate	Inappropriate	No opportunity to observe	Examples and comments
Verbal aspects				
A. Speech acts				
1. Speech act pair analysis				
2. Variety of speech acts				
B. Topic				
3. Selection				
4. Introduction				
5. Maintenance				
6. Change				
C. Turn taking				
7. Initiation				
8. Response				
9. Repair/revision				
10. Pause time				
11. Interruption/ overlap				
12. Feedback to speakers				
13. Adjacency				
14. Contingency				
15. Quantity/ conciseness				
D. Lexical selection/ use across speech acts				
16. Specificity/ accuracy				
17. Cohesion				
E. Stylistic variations				
18. The varying of communicative style				
Paralinguistic aspects				
F. Intelligibility and prosodics				
19. Intelligibility				
20. Vocal intensity				
21. Vocal quality				
22. Prosody				
23. Fluency				
Nonverbal aspects				
G. Kenesics and proxemics				
24. Physical proximity				
25. Physical contacts				
26. Body posture				
27. Foot/leg and hand/arm movements				
28. Gestures				
29. Facial expression				
30. Eye gaze				

Profile of Communicative Appropriateness (Penn, 1983)

Name _____   Features of sampling _____

Date _____   Unit of analysis _____

Person eliciting sample _____

		I	II	III	IV	V	VI	COMMENTS
Response to interlocutor	Request							
	Reply							
	Clarification request							
	Acknowledgement							
	Teaching probe							
	Others							
Control of semantic content	Topic initiation							
	Topic adherence							
	Topic shift							
	Lexical choice							
	Idea completion							
	Idea sequencing							
	Others							
Cohesion	Ellipsis							
	Tense use							
	Reference							
	Lexical substitution forms							
	Relative clauses							
	Prenominal adjectives							
	Conjunctions							
	Others							
Fluency	Interjections							
	Repetitions							
	Revisions							
	Incomplete phrases							
	False starts							
	Pauses							
	Word-finding difficulties							
	Others							
Sociolinguistic sensitivity	Polite forms							
	Reference to interlocutor							
	Placeholders, fillers, stereotypes							
	Acknowledgements							
	Self correction							
	Comment clauses							
	Sarcasm/humour							
	Control of direct speech							
	Indirect speech acts							
	Others							
Non-verbal communication	Vocal aspects: Intensity							
	Pitch							
	Rate							
	Intonation							
	Quality							
	Non-verbal aspects: Facial expression							
	Head movement							
	Body posture							
	Breathing							
	Social distance							
	Gesture and pantomime							
	Others							
	TOTALS							

Key:
I = Inappropriate; II = Mostly inappropriate; III = Some appropriate. IV = Mostly appropriate; V = Appropriate; VI = Could not evaluate

The Profile of Communicative Appropriateness.

7.3 Other Profiles

As we noted above, in the last few years there has been a big increase in the study of the relationship between pragmatics and disordered language. This can been seen, for example, in the work reported in Gallaher and Prutting (1983), Grunwell and James (1989), and McTear. and Conti-Ramsden (1989), as well as in numerous papers published in collections (for example Smith, 1988) and in the speech pathology journals (see McTear and Conti-Ramsden for accounts of some of these). Much of this work has been devoted to aspects of the assessment of pragmatics in the speech/language pathology clinic. As McTear and Conti-Ramsden (1989) have pointed out, these assessment procedures (as with other areas of linguistic inquiry) tend to fall into two broad categories: standardized tests, and 'pragmatic checklists' or profiles.

In clinical pragmatic assessment the main emphasis appears to have been on children with speech/language disorders. For example, Bates (1976) and McTear (1985) examine the acquisition of pragmatics by children, Smith (1988) concentrates her discussion on pragmatics in children, and many of the contributions to Gallaher and Prutting (1983) deal with speech/language disordered children. McTear and Conti-Ramsden (1989) provide a current bibliography of such work, including work of their own. Several profiles are noted in this literature as being designed for use with children: Roth and Spekman (1984a,b), McTear (1985), Bedrosian (1985), Prutting and Kirchner (1983, 1987, see above), Stickling (1987) and Dewart and Summers (1988). See also Long and Fey (1990a) for an account of a computerized pragmatic profile. It can be argued, of course, whether all of these are genuinely profiles, or whether they adopt too broad or too narrow a definition of pragmatics, but that is a discussion for elsewhere. We have also excluded from consideration other assessments of "functional ability" (e.g. FCP, Sarno, 1969; EFCP, Skinner, et al, 1984), although recognizing their link with current work.

The assessment of pragmatic abilities in aphasics is a relatively neglected area in comparison with the work on children. The Protocol of Prutting and Kirchner, which the authors note can be used both with children and with adults, and the Profile of Communicative Appropriateness, designed by Claire Penn (1988, see above) specifically for use with aphasics are exceptions.

Gerber and Gurland (1989) attempted a synthesis of the Pragmatic Protocol and the PCA for use with aphasic patients. Their APPLS (Assessment Protocol of Pragmatic-Linguistic Skills) is based on earlier pragmatic profiles (Gerber Wollner and Geller, 1982, Gurland, Chwat and Gerber Wollner, 1982), and aims to include both partners in the exchange rather than just the patient. It concentrates on turn-taking, and the breakdown of conversation and subsequent repair strategies. It avoids the use of the appropriate/inappropriate scoring technique, relying instead on noting where in the sample a particular problem occurred. This does leave, however, little room to record successful conversational turns (which have to be described verbally). A final qualitative summary also relies on verbal description. The overall impression of APPLS, then, is less like that of the other profiles we have investigated, and more like that of a guided written report. For this reason we have excluded it from our detailed look at pragmatic profiles.

Conclusion

The study of Ball *et al* (in press) demonstrated some of the problems involved in profiling areas of communication that are less concrete than many of the traditional concerns of clinical linguistics. It is clear from the data presented, that clinician training in pragmatic analysis is essential to avoid the discrepancies in inter-scorer reliability that were found. If everyone is recording the same behaviour in the same way, then a pragmatic profile is of worth, otherwise it can only be misleading.

Apart from topics such as interscorer reliability, further questions remain to be asked. Chief among them is the relative weighting of the parameters used in the profiles. If someone scores badly on fluency, is this more or less important than a good score on turn-taking? How useful are the sections on these charts - and should they too have a relative weighting. Are they relatable to remediation procedures, or simply constructs of the linguist? These questions, however, await further work.

Chapter 8

SOCIOLINGUISTICS AND BILINGUALISM

Introduction
This chapter will be dealing with two aspects of linguistics that have not traditionally featured in the testing or profiling literature: sociolinguistics and bilingualism. We will argue that both are important to an adequate analysis of patients' speech and language abilities, and that we can adapt some of the profiling techniques we have already examined for use in these areas.

8.1 Sociolinguistics
In his seminal work on clinical linguistics, Crystal (1981) discusses the possibility of the creation of a "clinical sociolinguistics" to complement the advances in other areas of clinical linguistics (a point he returns to in Crystal (1984)). In this discussion, Crystal gives the example of a clinical linguistic interaction between a clinician and a patient that illustrates the difference between discourse in clinical settings, and "natural" conversation.

Crystal acknowledges that this area of study might well come to be termed "clinical pragmatics" or "clinical discourse analysis" rather than "clinical sociolinguistics", and this is of course dealt with in the previous chapter.

In this chapter, therefore, we will exclude pragmatic and discourse related issues from our narrower definition of socio-linguistics. A further area of study that has been included under the label of sociolinguistics in some publications (see, for example, Trudgill, 1974a, Fasold, 1984, and Wardhaugh, 1986) is bi- or multilingualism and this is returned to in section 8.2 below. In this section we wish to concentrate on "core" areas of sociolinguistics, and see how they may be integrated into clinical linguistics.

By "core areas" of sociolinguistics in this account is meant the relation between language variation on the one hand, and non-linguistic features on the other. For the purposes of this chapter, the following non-linguistic features will be considered: social class, geographic region, sex, and age as aspects of speaker variability, and style as an aspect of environmental variability. We will examine these features in turn.

Speaker Variability
Social Class and Region
Social class membership and regional origin are linked socio-linguistically in many societies. For example, in Britain the higher up the social scale you are situated the fewer regional features of speech will be used. The non-regional R.P. pronunciation, and the non-regional Standard English dialect will be found with members of the upper middle classes, while localised accent (see Wells, 1982) and dialect features (see Trudgill and Chambers, 1991) will be encountered with members of the lower working class. In between in terms of class membership are found speakers whose accent and dialect will reflect some regional features, these decreasing with higher social class.

All of this is, of course, well known from the work of Labov (e.g. 1966, 1972), Trudgill (1974b, 1986) and others. It is also known that it is not a universal characteristic of speech communities that the link between class and region operates in this manner. Work referred to in Trudgill (1974a) shows that in India (for Kannaḍa) the higher the class (i.e. caste) the speaker is, the more likely they are to use regional forms, and the retention of standard, cross-regional forms is found with low caste speakers. Indeed, it has to be remembered that in bilingual situations, there may not be an equal spread of language users among all the social classes. As noted, for example, in Ball (1988c), in parts of Wales the Welsh speakers are restricted to lower class groups (for example in rural areas), or to professional middle class groups (in the metropolitan areas), and in this case a class analysis of speakers' language use is unhelpful.

We must now consider how important is the class/region feature of language variation in terms of the speech/language clinician. Considering only phonological disorders, it is comparatively easy to envisage a situation where aspects of class/regional variation in language can complicate an analysis. Assuming a patient presenting with a fricative simplification process, whereby target labio-dentals and interdentals are realised as labio-dentals, and target alveolars and palato-alveolars as alveolars, we might feel we have a relatively common and uncomplicated simplification of contrasts to deal with. However, if this patient originates from a region (such as London) where the merger of interdentals with labio-dentals is common, and from a class likely to use this feature, then this analysis must be challenged. It may well be that what we have here is simply a process affecting the alveolar vs. palato-alveolar contrast, with the loss of interdentals simply reflecting community norms.

Further, apart from issues of analysis, the planning of remediation programmes must be reconsidered. In the case noted above, serious consideration must be given as to whether training in the production of the contrast between interdental and labio-dental fricatives should be given, when such a contrast may not exist, or exist only peripherally in the patient's speech community.

Another case reported to me (J. Stephens, personal communication) involved a variable process of final consonant deletion. A clinician spent considerable time training the child involved to produce a final /s/ in the word "yes", while the child's mother produced nothing but "yeah" in answer to the clinician's questions!

One can imagine similar issues arising in a wide range of phonological and syntactic "disorders" from patients of different regional and class backgrounds. It is clearly important, in terms of any clinical sociolinguistics, that such issues can be identified, and remediation issues addressed.

Sex and Age

Researchers interested in the interaction of speaker's sex and linguistic variation have identified two broad approaches; what might be termed the "macro-linguistic" and the "micro-linguistic". The first of these is concerned with issues to do with discourse

105

(topic control, turn-taking, length of turn, feedback, tag questions, etc), politeness phenomena, use of expletives, and patriarchy in the lexicon (see Coates, 1986). The second follows more in the mold of the "classical Labovian" paradigm, and investigates the use of linguistic variables according to the sex of the speaker. While both of these areas are of interest to the interaction between clinician and patient, we will treat the first of these topics as outside the scope of "core" sociolinguistics as outlined above and concentrate on the second.

This again is important in terms of both analysis of speech/language disorders and their remediation. The research referred to in, for example, Trudgill (1974a,b) and Wardhaugh (1986), show that in general women are likely to use prestige forms of a linguistic variable more often than men. This clearly interacts with what we were examining above. Localised forms (such as the loss of contrast between interdental and labio-dental fricatives) may well be common in working class speakers; but further, how common they are may well depend on whether the speaker concerned is male or female. If we devise some means of noting these regional/class differences, this must be sensitive enough to note differences due to sex of the speaker.

Again, this does of course have implications for planning intervention. A particular linguistic feature may well be a marker of sex differences in a speech community, in that men use a particular variant most often while women use a different one. It is necessary, therefore, that such differences be integrated into remediation programmes: not necessarily an easy task.

Age of the speaker also often correlates with linguistic variation, in that certain variants of specific variables reflect older community speech norms, and so are retained by older speakers. This too is going to have an effect on both our understanding of a patient's linguistic output, and on the design of any treatment regime. An obvious example might be the retention by older R.P. speakers of yod in certain /#Cju-/ strings where it has been lost by younger speakers; e.g. "suit" /sjut/ ~ /sut/, "lute" /ljut/ ~ /lut/. Here, one has to be aware both that such pronunciations are perfectly acceptable for the older age group, and - if a general process of yod-deletion is found in the data of an older speaker - one has to decide whether to train just those yod clusters used by younger RP speakers, or to include the types noted above as well.

Environmental Variability.

By this term we mean what has been called "style" or "register" differences by other authors; that is to say variability of language caused by the degree of formality of the context of utterance. This in turn can depend on who the interlocutors are (and their comparative status), the topic of the conversation, and the circumstance of the conversation (e.g. casual conversation vs. an interview situation).

Clearly, such a feature is important for clinical linguistics, if only because so much of the data which is used for analysis is obtained in ways that are unusual to say the least in comparison with normal "casual" conversation. Even if we are moving away somewhat from relying solely on standardised tests utilising set language elicitation procedures, any form of speech collection is still non-normal in some way. This is because the normal context of utterance of the patient will be with family, friends, colleagues etc; not with speech/language clinicians.

This, therefore, may clearly have an effect on the reliability of the data collected. Indeed, one of the main interests of sociolinguistics has been in the methodology of data collection, in particular access to the vernacular (i.e. that style of speech that is subject to the least amount of monitoring by the speaker). The problem of gaining access to the vernacular has been termed "the observer's paradox": the goal of sociolinguists is to record the style of speech used by speakers when they are not being observed by outsiders, and the only way to achieve this is to observe them.

It may well be that the goal of clinical linguists is not necessarily the same, i.e. to record speech as used by speakers when not being observed by outsiders. Nevertheless, if all we can gain on occasions is a speech style radically different from that used by the speaker with their friends and family, then we are in great danger of making a false analysis of the linguistic repertoire and abilities normally open to the patient.

It might be expected that this false analysis will always err in the direction of underestimation of the patient's linguistic abilities. However, the converse is also found, in that patients can produce, under the extremely formalising context of the speech therapy clinic and perhaps of a formal test situation, phonological contrasts (for example) that they do not employ in casual speech.

Various methods have been employed by sociolinguists from Labov (1966) onwards to break out of the vicious circle of the observer's paradox and record examples of casual speech styles. These have involved questions designed to elicit emotional responses (through asking about dangerous or humorous episodes, or reminiscences), through verbal tasks involving the description of a non-linguistic event (such as Labov's "shoe-lace test", or the reporter's test of DeRenzi and Ferrari (1978)), to group work recording interactions between peers.

Not all of these will be appropriate within the clinic, as group interactions in particular may not be easy to set up, except when patients with similar disorders may be attending group sessions. This, however, is not the same as a group of friends/relatives which happens to include the patient. Nevertheless, techniques such as the reporter's test have clearly proved their use with certain patient types, and the emotive question may also prove helpful in breaking down any perceived "formality" in a patient's responses. Other techniques might involve the use of a formal test instrument, followed by a marked change in style by the therapist, who can leave a tape-recorder running, while giving the impression that the investigation is over. The resulting "small-talk" may well prove a good source of linguistic material, that is relatively informal in style, and could prove an adequate input for profiling techniques (see Crystal, 1982).

There is clearly a need for more research on how representative the data is that is collected for clinical analysis; a start on this is made when we recognize the fact that patients in the speech/language clinic are just as likely as anyone else to have, and to use, a wide range of linguistic styles.

Clinical Sociolinguistic Checklists.

We have shown above that the core areas of sociolinguistics are relevant to clinical linguistics. The problem remains of how they can be integrated into the analysis of disordered speech/language, and the subsequent remediation programmes, and whether devices like profiles are useful here.

Already, some current assessment procedures do make provision for language variation. For example, the phonology profile PROPH (see Crystal, 1982, and Chapter 3) has a line for the marking of accent conventions for a particular patient. However, this implies that such conventions are already known to the clinician; while most clinicians trained in phonetics and linguistics will be aware that such differences occur, it may not be so easy for them to gain quick and easy access to the material where such details are available.

However, to provide, for example, separate PROPH charts for every regional accent system within English (not considering variation due to other factors) would clearly not be feasible.

It might appear, then, that the integration of the core areas of sociolinguistics discussed above into clinical linguistic assessments is an impossible task. We suggest that this is not in fact so, and that steps can be taken in this direction without producing something too unwieldy to use. This would involve the construction of profile-like "clinical sociolinguistic checklists" (CSCs). Each CSC would be designed for a particular linguistic level, e.g. phonology, lexis, or syntax; further each would be designed for a particular patient selection, i.e. there would be no need to include information on British accents in a checklist designed for use in the U.S. In this respect, they would clearly not operate as profiles of individual patients, but as profiles of particular speech communities.

The CSC would contain information on differences from standard forms (i.e. R.P. for British phonology; or Standard English for syntax), and note what group of speaker (by class, region, sex, age etc), or context (formal vs. informal), or both would be likely to use the form in question. In this way clinicians could see at a glance whether it was likely (obviously one cannot make categorical statements in this regard) that the non-standard form used was sociolinguistically acceptable for the patient, or was more likely an example of disordered speech/language.

Clearly, the production of a whole range of CSCs for different linguistic levels and population groups would be a major undertaking, and we have not the space in this short chapter to produce such a set of checklists. However, to demonstrate the type of chart envisaged, we will conclude this section with an illustrative fragment of a phonology checklist for use in England (see also Ball, in press).

CLINICAL SOCIOLINGUISTIC CHECKLIST
PHONOLOGY (Base R.P.)

base variant	non-base vart	sociolinguistic detail
/θ/ ~ /ð/	/f/ ~ /v/	London; [C:X:S]
/θ/ ~ /ð/	[t̪] ~ [d̪]	S. Irish; [S]
[ɫ]	[l]	S. Wales, Newcastle; [C]
/Cju-/	/Cu-/	East Anglia; [C:X:S]
<Vr> = /V#/	/Vr/ = [ɹ]	West; part Lanc; [C]
<Vr> = /V#/	/Vr/ = [r/ɾ]	Scotland
/h/	Ø	maj Eng; S Wales; [C;X;S]
verb-ing	/ɪn/ ~ /ən/	all ex RP; [C;S]
/ʌ/	/ʊ/	Mid+N. Eng; [C]
/-ʊk/	/-uk/	Merseyside; [C]

Illustrative Fragment of a CSC for Phonology.
Key: C: class; X: sex; S: style.

8.2 Bilingualism

Interest in the bilingual speech/language disordered patient has been growing over the last decade. A major contribution in this area has been Miller's (1984) collection, and subsequent articles in the speech pathology journals. Bilingualism itself is, of course, not a problem (estimates vary, but it would seem that at least half, if not more, of the world's population is bi- or multilingual). The difficulty that arises with bilingual patients is how to conduct an adequate assessment of their linguistic abilities, and how to plan an adequate remediation programme bearing in mind that they operate with two (or more) languages, while the clinician may only operate with one.

We have only the space here to consider the first of these problems: how to assess the bilingual's linguistic abilities. What has to be remembered here is that we are not dealing with two monolinguals to be assessed as if a monolingual speaker of Language A, and a monolingual speaker of Language B. If we do this, we may well find that certain aspects of A or of B appear to be used differently from the way the monolingual speakers use them. In other words there may be interference (phonological, morphological, syntactic or lexical) from one language to another. This, however, should not be seen as an example of disordered speech or language, as it may well be the case that this is how the entire bilingual community use their languages. As an easy example, we can consider the Welsh speaker when speaking English in Britain, or the Spanish speaker speaking English in America: they clearly demonstrate accent features that are due to interference from their other language (Welsh, or Spanish). It is clearly no part of the speech pathologist's job to change these interference features as they constitute the accent of that group of speakers in the same way that a Yorkshire speaker or a New England speaker has an accent.

Unfortunately, not all bilingual speakers exhibit the same patterns of language dominance (so interference), and not all come from bilingual communities and so may have no norms of usage against which to compare. Nevertheless, many of the bilingual communities in Britain and the U.S. are fairly well established. In these cases, it may well be possible to construct assessment materials (such as profiles) that could take into account the full range of the speakers' linguistic repertoires (i.e. both languages) and the patterns of interference between the languages. Such a profile would naturally be quite complicated, and to date no comprehensive bilingual assessment instrument has been attempted. There have, however, been attempts at producing profiles for languages other than English; some of which can be used for minority languages (and so bilingual speakers) (see references in Ball, 1988b). In these cases it has to be remembered that we are, in fact, assessing monolingually (but twice). In some cases this is not such a problem, however. For some minority languages (such as the Celtic languages in Britain, or native American languages in the U.S.), there are no, or few, monolingual speakers left of the minority languages. Assessing the Welsh of a Welsh-language speaker, therefore, involves a comparison with other bilingual speakers, even if any assessment of their English is not comparing like with like.

We will conclude this section with a brief look at a syntax profile designed for use with Welsh speakers (from Ball, 1988b). The Chart designed to deal with this area (LLARSP, see charts at end of chapter) is, unlike LARSP for English, divided into three sub-charts. This reflects the different linguistic structure of the language, which has a rich system of inflectional morphology, and a grammatically important set of word-initial phonological changes ("mutations").

To cope with this, we have a syntax chart (LLARSP-C) which echoes to a great extent the categories and stages of LARSP. It is worth noting, however, that the clause patterns reflect the fact that the normal word-order in Welsh is VSO (verb-subject-object), and that the phrase level patterns reflect the fact that adjectives follow the noun.

The second chart is the morphology chart (LLARSP-M), and this is divided into sections for noting what use (and what errors) is made of inflections on verbs, nouns, prepositions and adjectives. Again, a particular feature of the language is shown in the fact that many prepositions take personal endings.

112

The final chart is the "mutations" chart (LLARSP-T). This has sections to show the patterns of usage of the mutations, divided into their three main types, and in their different grammatical contexts. This chart also allows the noting of errors of various types with these mutations.

Clearly, then, profiles for different languages may differ considerably from the patterns we have seen for English in earlier chapters. Many languages (such as Chinese) make use of pitch differences to mark differences at the word level ("tone"). This would require a radically different type of profile from PROP for English. Some languages, such as Finnish and Turkish, are morphologically agglutinative: that is to say that a number of suffixes can be added on to word stems to add extra meaning, leading to long complicated word structures. Clearly, a morphological profile would be important for this type of language.

It is to be hoped that profiles for many languages and for many linguistic aspects will be developed in the future, as an aid to assessment and to remediation.

The Clinician's Guide to Linguistic Profiling

Name		Age		Sample date		Type	

A	**Unanalysed**			**Problematic**			
	1 Unintelligible	2 Symbolic Noise	3 Deviant	1 Incomplete	2 Ambiguous	3 Stereotypes	

	Code-Switching				
	1 Sentence	2 Clause	3 Element	4 Phrasal	

B Responses

	Stimulus type	Totals	Repetition	Normal Response								Abnormal	
				Major								Structural	θ	Problems
				Elliptical			Reduced	Full	Minor				
				1	2	3+							
	Questions												
	Others												

C Spontaneous

D Reactions

		General	Structural	θ	Other	Problems

Stage I

Minor		Responses		Vocatives	Other		Problems
Major	Comm	Quest	Statement				
	'V'	'Q'	'V'	'N'	other		problems

Stage II

Conn		Clause				Phrase	
	VX	QX	VS	AX		DN	VV
			SO	VO		NAdj	Vpart
			SC	VC		NN	IntX
	paid X		NegX	other		PrN	Asp*yn*
						Cp.*yn*	Other

Stage III

X + S:NP		X + V:VP		X + C:NP	X + O:NP	X + A:AP	
VXY	QXY	VSO	VcSC	VOA	DNAdj		DND
paid	VS(X)	VSA	CVcS	VCA	NAdjAdj	Pron°	Cop
X Y		VSC	VcSA		PrDN	Aux¹	Asp
*gad*XY		NegXY		other	NDN		other

Stage IV

XY + S:NP		XY + V:VP		XY + C:NP	XY + O:NP	XY + A:AP	
VXY +	QXY +	VSAA	VcSXY		NPPrNP	VNeg	
paid	VSX(Y +)	VSOA	CVcSA		PrDNAdj	NegX	
XY +	tag	VSOC			NPDNP	2Aux	
		VSCA			cX		
		AAXY		other	XcX		other

Stage V

a	Coord	Coord	Coord	1		1 +	Postmod	1		1 +
c			SubordA	1		1 +	clause			
s	other	other	S	C	0					
other			Comparative				Postmod phrase	1 +		

(+)			(−)	

Stage VI

NP	VP	Clause	Conn	Clause			Phrase				
Initiator	complex	*cael*	a	Element θ	NP			Aux°θ	VP Aux¹θ	Aspθ	
		passive	c		D	Pr	Pron				
Coord.		complem.		⇄ Concord	Dθ	Prθ		Aux°	Aux		
			s		D⇄	Pr⇄		Cop			
		exclam.			Gen	Cp.*yn*					
Other							Ambiguous				

Stage VII

Discourse		Syntactic comprehension	
A Connectivity	empty *mae'n*		
Comment Clause	empty *mae 'na*	Style	
Emphatic order	other		

Total No. Sentences	Mean No. Sentences Per Turn	Mean Sentence Length

© D. Crystal, P. Fletcher, M. Garman, 1981 revision, University of Reading
© Martin J. Ball, Welsh version

The LLARSP-C chart.

Name	Age	Sample date	Type

	Morphology	Errors

BOD

	mae 1	mae + neg 1	mae + Q 1	mae + indef:	
	2	2	2	*does*	person
	3	3	3	*oes?*	
	1	1	1	emphatic:	
	2	2	2	*ydy/sydd*	form
VP	3	3	3	deictic:	
				dyma/dyna	

	oedd 1	Bu 1	bydd 1	byddai 1	buasai 1	tense
	2	2	2	2	2	
	3	3	3	3	3	
	1	1	1	1	1	person
	2	2	2	2	2	
	3	3	3	3	3	

imperative sing: plur: Other

V reg

-th 1	-odd 1		
2	2	imperative sing	tense
3	3	plur:	
1	1		
2	2	Other	person
3	3		

V irreg

gwneud	cael	mynd	dod	
1 1	1 1	1 1	1 1	
2 2	2 2	2 2	2 2	tense
3 3	3 3	3 3	3 3	
1 1	1 1	1 1	1 1	
2 2	2 2	2 2	2 2	person
3 3	3 3	3 3	3 3	
			imp. s	
			imp. p	

Other

Responses

ydw	ydy	oes	oedd	do	gwnaf	ie	other	pos/neg
nac	nac	nac	nac	naddo	na	nage		type

NP	Plural:	-au	-iau	-ion/on	-i -od	θ
		V→V	V→V-au	V→V-iau	V→V-ion/on	form
		other				y→yr
	Sing:	-en/yn		Det: y yr 'r		yr→y

Prep	class 1 (-o/i)	1 2 3 1 2 3	θ
	class 2 (-ddo/ddi)	1 2 3 1 2 3	person
	gan	1 2 3 1 2 3	class

Adj	feminine			Other	θ
	comparison	-ach	-af		θ
					form

Summary	Total Infl. Morphemes	No. Types	Type:Token ratio	Types/categ. VP NP Prep Adj	Total Errors VP NP Prep Adj

The LLARSP-M chart.

| | Name | | Age | | Sample date | | Type | |

	Context	+ SM	Rad	Context	+ SM	Rad
SM	Pr + N D + Nf Num + N Poss + N/V *dyma/dyna* + N			Nf + Adj yn + N/Adj V + O (part) + V Other		

	Context	+ NM		rad	+ SM	
NM	*fy* + N/V *yn* + Nproper *yn* + N Other					

	Context	+ AM		rad	+ SM	
AM	*ei* + N/V *a* + N Other					

over-mutation	SM
	NM
	AM

| Other | |

© 1987 Martin J. Ball

The LLARSP-T chart.

Anthony, A., Bogle, D., Ingram, T. and McIsaac, M. (1971) *The Edinburgh Articulation Test*. Edinburgh: Livingstone.

Baker-van den Goorbergh, L. (1990) Computerised Language Error Analysis Report. *Clinical Linguistics & Phonetics*, 4, 285-93.

Baker-van den Goorbergh, L. and Baker, K. (1991) *CLEAR. Computerised Language Error Analysis Report*. Manual and software. Kibworth, Leics.: Far Communications.

Ball, M. J. (1988a) Clinical linguistic encounters. *Clinical Linguistics & Phonetics*, 2, 143-51.

Ball, M. J. (1988b) LARSP to LLARSP: the design of a grammatical profile for Welsh. *Clinical Linguistics & Phonetics*, 2, 55-73.

Ball, M. J. (Ed.) (1988c) *The Use of Welsh*. Clevedon: Multilingual Matters.

Ball, M. J. (1989) *Phonetics for Speech Phonology*. London: Taylor & Francis/Whurr.

Ball, M. J. (1991) Recent developments in the transcription of non-normal speech. *Journal of Communication Disorders*, 24, 59-78.

Ball, M. J. (in press) Is a clinical sociolinguistics possible? *Clinical Linguistics & Phonetics*, 6.

Ball, M. J., Davies, E., Duckworth, M. and Middlehurst, R. (in press) Assessing the assessments: a comparison of two clinical pragmatic profiles. *Journal of Communication Disorders*.

Bates, E. (1976) *Language and Context: the Acquisition of Pragmatics*. New York: Academic Press.

Bedrosian, J. (1985) An approach to developing conversational competence. In Ripich, D. and Spinelli, F. (eds), *School Discourse Problems*. London: Taylor and Francis.

Bloom, L. and Lahey, M. (1978) *Language Development and Language Disorders*. New York: John Wiley and Sons.

Brown, R. (1973) *A First Language: the early stages*. Cambridge Mass.: Harvard University Press.

Chapman, R. (1981) Computing mean length of utterance in

morphemes. In Miller, J. F.

Clark, J. and Yallop, C. (1990) *An Introduction to Phonetics and Phonology*. Oxford: Blackwell.

Coates, J. (1986) *Woman, Men and Language*. London: Longman.

Code, C. and Ball, M. J. (1982) Fricative production in Broca's aphasia: a spectrographic analysis. *Journal of Phonetics*, **10**, 325-31.

Code, C. and Ball, M. J. (Eds.) (1984) *Experimental Clinical Phonetics*. London: Croom Helm.

Compton, A. and Hutton, J. (1978) *Compton-Hutton Phonological Assessment*. San Francisco, CA.: Carousel House.

Crystal, D. (1979) *Working with LARSP*. London: Edward Arnold.

Crystal, D. (1981) *Clinical Linguistics*. Vienna: Springer-Verlag.

Crystal, D. (1982) *Profiling Linguistic Disability*. London: Edward Arnold.

Crystal, D. (1984) *Linguistic Encounters with Language Handicap*. Oxford: Blackwell.

Crystal, D., Fletcher, P. and Garman, M. (1976) *The Grammatical Analysis of Language Disability*. London: Edward Arnold.

Crystal, D., Fletcher, P. and Garman, M. (1989) *The Grammatical Analysis of Language Disability*. 2nd edition. London: Whurr.

Dalton, P. and Hardcastle, W. J. (1977) *Disorders of Fluency and their effects on communication*. London: Edward Arnold.

DeRenzi, E. and Ferrari, C. (1978) The reporter's test: a sensitive test to detect expressive disturbances in aphasics. *Cortex*, **14**, 279-93.

Dewart, H. and Summers, S. (1988) *The Pragmatics Profile of Early Communication Skills*. Windsor: NFER-Nelson.

Duckworth, M., Allen, G., Hardcastle, W. and Ball, M. J. (1990) Extensions to the International Phonetic Alphabet for the transcription of atypical speech. *Clinical Linguistics and Phonetics*, **4**, 273-80.

Elbert, M. and Gierut, J. (1986) *Handbook of Clinical Phonology*. London: Taylor and Francis.

Fasold, R. (1984) *The Sociolinguistics of Society.* Oxford: Blackwell.

Gallaher, T. and Prutting, C. (eds) (1983) *Pragmatic Assessment and Intervention Issues in Language.* San Diego: College Hill.

Gerber, S. and Gurland, G. B. (1989) Applied pragmatics in the assessment of aphasia. *Seminars in Speech and Language,* **10,** 263-81.

Gerber Wollner, S. and Geller, E. (1982) Methods of assessing pragmatic abilities. In Irwin, J. (Ed.), *Pragmatics: the role in Language Development.* LaVerne, CA: Fox Point Publishing Ltd.

Goldman, R. and Fristoe, M. (1972) *Test of Articulation.* Circle Pines, Minn.: American Guidance Service Inc.

Grunwell, P. (1982) *Clinical Phonology.* London: Croom Helm.

Grunwell, P. (1985) PACS. Phonological Assessment of Child Speech. Windsor: NFER-Nelson.

Grunwell, P. (1987) *Clinical Phonology.* 2nd edition. London: Croom Helm.

Grunwell, P. (1988) Phonological assessment, evaluation and explanation of speech disorders in children. *Clinical Linguistics & Phonetics,* **2,** 221-52.

Grunwell, P. and James, A. (eds) (1989) *The Functional Evaluation of Language Disorders.* London: Croom Helm.

Gurland, G. B., Chwat, S. E. and Gerber Wollner, S. (1982) Establishing a communication profile in adult aphasia: analysis of communicative acts and conversational sequences. In Brookshire, R. (Ed.), *Clinical Aphasiology Conference Proceedings.* Minneapolis: BRK Publishers.

Hodson, B. (1980) *The Assessment of Phonological Processes.* Danville, Ill.: Interstate Inc.

Ingram, D. (1976) *Phonological Disability in Children.* London: Edward Arnold.

Ingram, D. (1981) *Procedure for the Phonological Analysis of Children's Language.* Baltimore, MD.: University Park Press.

IPA (1989) Report on the 1989 Kiel Convention. *Journal of the International Phonetic Association,* **19,** 67-80.

Jassem, W. (1990) Review of 'Longman Pronunciation Dictionary' (John Wells). *Phonetica,* **47,** 244-47.

Labov, W. (1966) *The Social Stratification of English in New York City.* Washington D.C.: Center for Applied Linguistics.

Labov, W. (1972) *Sociolinguistic Patterns.* Oxford: Blackwell.

Laver, J. (1980) *The Phonetic Description of Voice Quality.* Cambridge: Cambridge University Press.

Lee, L. (1974) *Developmental Sentence Analysis.* Evanston, Ill.: Northwestern University Press.

Leech, G. (1983) *Principles of Pragmatics.* London: Longmans.

Levinson, S. (1983) *Pragmatics.* Cambridge: Cambridge University Press.

Long, S. H. (1987) "Computerized profiling" of clinical language samples. *Clinical Linguistics & Phonetics,* **1,** 97-105.

Long, S. H. and Fey, M. (1990a) Language sample analysis with the Macintosh. Poster presented at the American Speech-Language-Hearing Association Annual Convention, Seattle, Washington, 1990.

Long, S. H. and Fey, M. (1990b) Reciprocal use of SALT and *Computerized Profiling.* Poster presented at the American Speech-Language-Hearing Association Annual Convention, Seattle, Washington, 1990.

Long, S. H. and Long, S. T. (1990) Computer-assisted instruction (CAI) for LARSP profiling. Poster presented at the American Speech-Language-Hearing Association Annual Convention, Seattle, Washington, 1990.

Lund, N. and Duchan, J. (1987) *Assessing Children's Language in Naturalistic Contexts.* 2nd edition. Englewood Cliffs, NJ: Prentice-Hall.

McReynolds, L. and Engmann, D. (1976) *Distinctive Feature Analysis of Misarticulations.* Baltimore, MD.: University Park Press.

McTear, M. (1985) *Children's Conversations.* Oxford: Blackwell.

McTear, M. and Conti-Ramsden, G. (1989) Assessment of pragmatics. In Grundy, K. (1989) *Linguistics in Clinical Practice.* London: Taylor and Francis.

Miller, J. F. (1981) *Assessing language Production in Children:*

Experimental Procedures. Baltimore, MD.: University Park Press.

Miller, J. F. and Chapman, R. (1985) *SALT: Systematic Analysis of Language Transcripts.* User's guide and software. Madison, Wisc.: Language Analysis Lab, Waisman Center on Mental Retardation and Human Development, University of Wisconsin.

Miller, N. (Ed.) (1984) *Bilingualism and Language Disability.* London: Croom Helm.

Müller, D., Munro, S. and Code, C. (1981) *Language Assessment for Remediation.* London: Croom Helm.

O'Connor, J. D. and Arnold, G. (1973) *Intonation of Colloquial English.* 2nd edition. London: Longmans.

Paul, R. (1981) Analyzing complex sentence development. In Miller, J. F.

Penn, C. (1983) *Syntactic and Pragmatic Aspects of Aphasic Language.* Unpublished doctoral thesis, University of the Witwatersrand.

Penn, C. (1988) The profiling of syntax and pragmatics in aphasia. *Clinical Linguistics & Phonetics,* 2, 179-207.

Pollock, K. and Hall, P. (1991) An analysis of the vowel misarticulations of five children with developmental apraxia of speech. *Clinical Linguistics & Phonetics,* **5,** 207-24.

Pollock, K. and Keiser, N. (1990) An examination of vowel errors in phonologically disordered children. *Clinical Linguistics & Phonetics,* **4,** 161-78.

PRDS (1980) The phonetic representation of disordered speech. *British Journal of Disorders of Communication,* **15,** 217-23.

PRDS (1983) *The Phonetic Representation of Disordered Speech: Final Report.* London: The King's Fund.

Prutting, C. and Kirchner, D. (1983) Applied pragmatics. In Gallaher, T. and Prutting, C. (eds).

Prutting, C. and Kirchner, D. (1987) A clinical appraisal of the pragmatic aspects of language. *Journal of Speech and Hearing Disorders,* 52, 105-19.

Pye, C. (1987) *PAL: Pye Analysis of Language.* Manual and software. 200 Arrowhead Drive, Lawrence, Kansas 66049.

The Clinician's Guide to Linguistic Profiling

Pye, C. and Ingram, D. (1988) Automating the analysis of child phonology. *Clinical Linguistics & Phonetics,* **2,** 115-37.

Roth, F. and Spekman, N. (1984a) Assessing the pragmatic ability of children: Part 1. Organizational framework and assessment parameters. *Journal of Speech and Hearing Disorders,* 49, 2-11.

Roth, F. and Spekman, N. (1984b) Assessing the pragmatic ability of children: Part 2. Guidelines, considerations, and specific evaluation procedures. *Journal of Speech and Hearing Disorders,* 49, 12-17.

Sarno, M. (1969) *The Functional Communication Profile.* New York: New York University Medical Center.

Shriberg, L. (1986) *PEPPER: Programs to Examine Phonetic and Phonologic Evaluation Records.* Hillsdale, NJ.: Lawrence Erlbaum.

Shriberg, L. and Kent, R. D. (1982) *Clinical Phonetics.* New York: Macmillan.

Shriberg, L. and Kwiatkowski, J. (1980) *Natural Process Analysis (NPA).* New York: John Wiley.

Shriberg, L., Kwiatkowski, J. and Rasmussen, C. (1989a) *The Prosody-Voice Screening Profile (PVSP): I. Description and psychometric studies.* Paper presented at the American Speech-Language-Hearing Association Annual Convention, St Louis, Missouri, 1989.

Shriberg, L., Kwiatkowski, J. and Rasmussen, C. (1989b) *The Prosody-Voice Screening Profile (PVSP): II. Reference data and construct validity.* Paper presented at the American Speech-Language-Hearing Association Annual Convention, St Louis, Missouri, 1989.

Shriberg, L. and Lof, G. (1991) Reliability studies in broad and narrow transcription. *Clinical Linguistics & Phonetics,* **5,** 225-79.

Skinner, C., Wirz, S., Thompson, I. and Davidson, J. (1984) *Edinburgh Functional Communication Profile.* Buckingham: Winslow Press.

Smith, R. (1988) Pragmatics and speech pathology. In Ball, M. J. (ed), *Theoretical Linguistics and Disordered Language.*

London: Croom Helm.

Stickler, K. R. (1987) *Guide to Analysis of Language Transcripts*. Eau Claire, WI.: Thinking Publications.

Stoel-Gammon, C. and Dunn, C. (1985) *Normal and Disordered Phonology in Children*. Baltimore, MD.: University Park Press.

Stoel-Gammon, C. and Beckett Herrington, P. (1990) Vowel systems of normally developing and phonologically disordered children. *Clinical Linguistics & Phonetics, 4*, 145-60.

Trudgill, P. (1974a) *Sociolinguistics: An Introduction*. Harmondsworth: Penguin.

Trudgill, P. (1974b) *The Social Differentiation of English in Norwich*. Cambridge: Cambridge University Press.

Trudgill, P. (1986) *Dialects in Contact*. Oxford: Blackwell.

Trudgill, P. and Chambers, J. K. (Eds.) (1991) *Dialects of English*. London: Longmans.

Tyack, D. and Gottsleben, R. (1974) *Language Sampling, Analysis and Training: A Handbook for Teachers and Clinicians*. Palo Alto, Calif.: Consulting Psychologists Press.

Vierregge, W. H. (1987) Basic aspects of phonetic segmental transcription. *Zeitschrift für Dialektologie und Linguistik Beihefte, 54*, 5-55.

Wardhaugh, R. (1986) *An Introduction to Sociolinguistics*. Oxford: Blackwell.

Weiner, F. (1979) *Phonological Process Analysis (PPA)*. Baltimore, MD.: University Park Press.

Wells, J. (1982) *Accents of English*. (3 volumes). Cambridge: Cambridge University Press.

INDEX

articulation test 1, 12-5
ASS/CSD 69-72
bilingualism 10, 111-6
clause elements 60-8
Clinical Sociolinguistic
    Checklist 109-10
communicative metric 28, 33
computer profiling 36, 73-4,
    101
consonant clusters 26-7, 35
developmental metric 3, 25,
    28, 33, 35-6, 62-72,
    88-94
distinctive features 24, 27-
    8, 33, 44
error analysis 23
generative phonology 44
intonation 45-50
LARSP 59-68
LLARSP 114-6
length 12
levels of analysis
lexis 4, 9, 75, 76-9
loudness 45, 50, 52
MLU 56-9, 69, 74
morphology 4, 6-9, 55, 56-9
PACS 33-44
PCA 97-8 100
phone 11, 34
  contrastive 35
phoneme 11, 23, 34
phonetics 4-6, 11-22
  phonetic symbols 12, 19-22
  segmental 11

suprasegmental 11
transcription 15-8, 33-4
phonology 4-6
  processes 24, 28, 35, 44
  segmental 23-44
  suprasegmental 45-54
phonotactics 24-5, 35
phrase elements 60-8
pitch 12, 45-6
pragmatics 10, 95-102
Pragmatic Protocol 96-7, 99
profiles 1-3, *passim*
PRISM-G 92-4
PRISM-L 80-7
PROP 46-50
PROPH 25-32
PROVOQ 50-4
semantics 4, 9, 75-94
  grammatical 75, 79, 88-94
  lexical 75, 76-87
sociolinguistics 10, 103-10
stress 12, 45
syntax 4, 6-9, 55-6
  clause level 60-8
  phrase level 60-8
  sentence level 60-8, 72
tempo 45, 50, 52
tests 1-2
variability 104-8
  environmental 107-8
  speaker 104-7
voice quality 12, 45-6, 50-4
vowels 26, 34
word level 60-8